PLEASURE AND INSTINCT

Founded by C. K. Ogden

The International Library of Psychology

PHYSIOLOGICAL PSYCHOLOGY
In 10 Volumes

PLEASURE AND INSTINCT

A Study in the Psychology of Human Action

A H BURLTON ALLEN

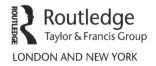

LONDON AND NEW YORK

First published in 1930
by Routledge, Trench, Trubner & Co., Ltd.
2 Park Square, Milton Park, Abingdon, Oxfordshire OX14 4RN
711 Third Avenue, New York, NY 10017

First issued in paperback 2014

Routledge is an imprint of the Taylor and Francis Group, an informa business

© 1930 A H Burlton Allen

All rights reserved. No part of this book may be reprinted or reproduced
or utilized in any form or by any electronic, mechanical, or other means,
now known or hereafter invented, including photocopying
and recording, or in any information storage or retrieval system, without
permission in writing from the publishers.

The publishers have made every effort to contact authors/copyright holders
of the works reprinted in the *International Library of Psychology*.
This has not been possible in every case, however, and we would
welcome correspondence from those individuals/companies
we have been unable to trace.

These reprints are taken from original copies of each book. In many cases
the condition of these originals is not perfect. The publisher has gone to
great lengths to ensure the quality of these reprints, but wishes to point
out that certain characteristics of the original copies will, of necessity, be
apparent in reprints thereof.

British Library Cataloguing in Publication Data
A CIP catalogue record for this book
is available from the British Library

Pleasure and Instinct
ISBN 0415-21072-0
Physiological Psychology: 10 Volumes
ISBN 0415-21131-X
The International Library of Psychology: 204 Volumes
ISBN 0415-19132-7

ISBN 13: 978-1-138-87546-3 (pbk)
ISBN 13: 978-0-415-21072-0 (hbk)

CONTENTS

PART I

PART II

SENSORY PLEASURE AND UNPLEASURE

v

PART III

PLEASURE AND UNPLEASURE IN RELATION TO THE MAIN INSTINCTS

scription of the development of self-assertive pride in the individual in normal life of society. There is no primitive instinct of submission co-ordinate with the impulse to dominance. The question whether self-assertion always originates from experiences of inferiority.

Early appearance of altruistic acts in children. Sentiments of love towards persons or groups of persons appear in order in the course of individual development, i.e. towards parents, towards equals and comrades, towards the conjugal partner and towards children. Devotion to the group and to wider classes, e.g. humanity. Review of the theory which regards all the forms of altruistic love as derived from the parental instinct. Reasons for rejecting this theory. Further consideration of the gregarious instinct. It involves a satisfaction in the presence of comrades living and in normal health ; and thus, when intellect is sufficiently developed, it must lead normally to the effort to maintain their lives and assist them when in distress. Gregariousness appears as a primitive instinct in man. Sympathy does not in itself lead to altruistic action ; the part it plays is to give additional warmth and insight to the impulse towards assistance of others, connected with gregariousness. The conclusion is that there is in man a fundamental impulse to join himself as a member to a larger group and to forward the interests of that group. This impulse shows itself also in the form of the family affections. Such an impulse tends naturally to expand into a devotion to the widest group of which a man can consider himself a member. It is consistent with the maintenance of the consciousness of separate personality. A likeness is found herein to mystical religious experiences.

The conclusion is that the original instinctive equipment of man consists in (1) the bodily self-maintaining process, including propagation, with a number of separate impulses developed as subsidiary to it, (2) the two " spiritual " impulses, of self-maximation and self-giving, (3) fear and anger, as reactions safeguarding the other instincts.

Pleasure does not lie only in the attainment of ends, the striving towards which is essentially unpleasant. Life is made up of conative trains which may be pleasant throughout, if progressing normally towards their end points. Entirely neutral states do not exist. Unpleasure follows on frustration of instinct, and is the result of conflict due to the persistence of the thwarted instinct. Relaxation to a lower level of activity is sometimes pleasant ; the case of narcotics.

The difficulty as to whether æsthetic satisfaction is dependent on the success of conation. Æsthetic satisfaction is

functioning. It is suggested that there are values attached : (1) to the success or non-success of conations, i.e. pleasure and unpleasure, (2) to the degrees of mental activity and passivity, in respect of which we feel ourselves more or less self-directed, (3) to the degrees of depth or intensity with which the self is engaged in a reaction. There are two other forms of the mental life, i.e. that which moves in the dimension between tension and relaxation, and that of degrees of unity. But to neither of these as such does felt value appear to be attached. There are no mixed feelings in the sense of a blending of positive and negative values. When feelings are simultaneous there tends to be a summation of similar values, whether positive or negative; and a relation of contradiction between positive and negative values. It is admitted that in the above the peculiar value attributed to " self-giving " is not fully explained. The relation of the other sorts of value to action is similar to that already described for pleasure.

PLEASURE & INSTINCT

A STUDY IN THE PSYCHOLOGY OF HUMAN ACTION

PART I
INTRODUCTORY

SUMMARY OF PRINCIPAL THEORIES OF PLEASURE AND
UNPLEASURE. QUESTIONS OF NOMENCLATURE

In the present work an attempt is made in the first place to define the nature of " feeling ", that which in ordinary language is called " pleasure and pain ", or in more technically psychological terms " the affective side of the mental life ". In the present state of psychology, however, there being little enough agreement on general principles, it is practically impossible to treat any one part of the mental life as a closed-off department, separate from the rest. This is particularly the case in regard to the feelings, and we shall in the course of our enquiry find ourselves carried on to consider a somewhat wide range of general psychological questions, particularly those connected with instinct.

Let us begin by giving a summary of the more important views hitherto held on the nature of pleasure and pain (or as we shall usually say) " unpleasure ". It is impossible to attempt to be exhaustive. We can only indicate the chief types of theory. Theories we shall find fall into two main classes : (1) those which consider the feelings an order of mental facts different in kind to sensations, to the cognitive elements of mind ; and related to the *form* of the psycho-physical process ; (2) those which treat them as essentially akin to sensation and having their own organs or brain-centre.

Under (1) there is in the first place the school which we may consider as deriving from Butler, who maintained that the primary fact is the existence in man of particular passions and appetites, but that pleasure or unpleasure arise according as these are successful or unsuccessful. " The very idea of interest or happiness consists in this, that an appetite or affection enjoys its object."[1] As the chief modern representatives of this view we may mention Stout and McDougall. It follows logically from it that these feelings must be held to appertain to the subjective side of the mental life, to be modifications of the self-state, arising in a secondary or epi-phenomenal manner in dependence on the course of conative activity.

The Hedonist school holds, it is true, that the relation of feeling to conation is the reverse of that first mentioned, i.e. it believes that conation and desire are determined by pleasure, not that pleasure is dependent on the result of conation. Yet this school does appear to hold that the connection between feeling and conation is necessary and indissoluble. For Mill has stated that desiring a thing and finding it pleasant, aversion to it and thinking of it as painful, are two parts of the same phenomenon,[2] and Spencer that for the word pleasure we can substitute the equivalent phrase—a feeling which we seek to bring into consciousness and retain there, and for the word pain, the equivalent phrase—a feeling which we seek to get out of consciousness and keep out.[3] Further, the adherents of this school do, it would seem, agree generally that pleasure and unpleasure are facts of the mental life which arise in dependence on the *form* of the psycho-physical process, i.e. are not independent mental facts of the same order as the cognitive elements of consciousness. This at least would appear to be involved in Herbert

---

[1] Butler, " Preface to Sermons ", Selby & Bigge, *British Moralists*, I, 192.

[2] See *Utilitarianism*, c. IV.

[3] *Principles of Psychology*, I, 280.

Spencer's view that pleasure is the concomitant of medium activities, beneficial to the organism, and pain the concomitant of either excessive or deficient activity, injurious to the organism ;[1] and we may find the same exemplified in the two principles stated by Bain, i.e. firstly that pleasure is connected with an increase and pain with an abatement of some or all of the vital functions, and secondly that pleasure accompanies the moderate discharge of nervous activity up to a point not exceeding the powers of reparation possessed by the organism.[2]

There are a number of other theories which agree in general that pleasure is the accompaniment of successful or easy vital activity, but endeavour to define the neural conditions more accurately. Lehmann in his elaborate work on the feelings gives the view that unpleasure occurs when the capacity for work of a nerve centre is lowered by its activity, and that pleasure accompanies an activity of the neurone which takes place without decrease of the capacity for work, but is greater according as the activity is greater ; or in other words unpleasure occurs when dissimilation is greater than assimilation, and pleasure occurs when they balance, but pleasure is greater according as both factors, assimilation and dissimilation, are greater.[3] According to Marshall pleasure occurs whenever the stimulus affecting an organ occasions the use of surplus stored force, unpleasure when the stored force is insufficient to the demands of the stimulus.[4] Störring holds a view closely similar to this.[5] Many more recent physiological theories agree in relating pleasure and unpleasure to the form or pattern of the neural activity. J. C. Herrick writes as follows : " The normal discharge then of definitely elaborated nervous circuits resulting in free unrestrained activity is pleasurable, in so far as the reaction comes into consciousness at all (of course, a large

---

[1] *Id.*, I, 272–9.
[2] Bain, *Senses and Intellect*, 303–17.
[3] Lehmann, *Die Hauptgesetze des menschlichen Gefühlslebens*, esp. 163–8.
[4] *Pain, Pleasure and Æsthetics*, 204 and 324.
[5] *Psychologie des menschlichen Gefühlslebens*, 70–72.

proportion of such reactions are strictly reflex and have no conscious significance). Conversely the impediment to such discharge, no matter what the occasion, results in a stasis in the nerve centres, the summation of stimuli and the development of a situation of unrelieved nervous tension which is unpleasant, until the tension is relieved by the appropriate adaptive reaction."[1] The view of W. M. Marston is similar to this, but he lays stress on the consciousness going with motor impulse, and finds the essence of pleasure and unpleasure in consciousness of mutual facilitation or antagonism between motor impulses.[2] W. B. Cannon has suggested that feeling is the result of certain patterns or combinations of neural activity (occurring it is true only in sub-cortical centres), which fix certain forms of reaction and bodily posture.[3]

(2) We have now to contrast with the foregoing those theories in which pleasure and unpleasure are assimilated to sensations, i.e. to the cognative contents of the mind. Of these we can distinguish two classes : (a) those which regard these feelings as organic sensations or complexes of such sensations, (b) those which regard them as mental elements distinct from other sensations but of the same order, and as arising from the excitation of a separate " feeling centre " in the brain. As an example of (a) we may take the following statement by R. B. Perry : " Feeling can be regarded as a sensory experience referred vaguely and diffusely to the body itself and immediately initiating responses of prolongation or rejection. Feeling in the broadest sense is any organic sensory complex in proportion as it is immediate and non-discriminatory. Feeling in the narrower sense in which it is associated with the duality of pleasure and pain is any such sensory complex, together with the interest taken in it for its own sake. Pleasures are non-discriminatory organic sensations which are immediately liked, pains

---

[1] Herrick, *Introduction to Neurology* (1927), 298.
[2] Marston, *Emotions of Normal People*, chapter V.
[3] W. B. Cannon in *Feelings and Emotions* (Wittenberg Symposium), 266–7.

non-discriminatory organic sensations, immediately dis-
liked."[1] He would apparently hold that the acts of
prolongation or rejection are reflexes which in the course
of evolution have been established in relation to favourable or unfavourable bodily conditions.

The theory of the " sensational " nature of pleasure
and unpleasure is, however, more often held in the form
(b). We may take Stumpf as giving a clear version of this.[2]
He has maintained that sensory pleasure and pain are
in fact sensations. As such they can exist independently
of other sensations (e.g. cutaneous or internal pain).
But in the case of many of the senses, especially sight,
touch, and hearing they are excited through the medium
of those sense organs, and therefore only exist as " Mit "
or " Annexe-Empfindungen ".[3] In both cases a feeling-
centre is involved, in the one class affected direct, in the
other through medium of the other senses. They belong,
therefore, not to the subjective (zuständlich) part of
consciousness, but to the objective (gegenständlich), not
to the functions, but to the matter of consciousness, in
the same way as colours, sounds, etc., are reckoned.[4]
There is therefore no necessary connection between these
" feeling sensations " and conation. They do in fact
constitute the primary motives of accepting or rejecting
behaviour,[5] but Stumpf's explanation why this should be
so is not very clear ; apparently he would hold that somehow in point of fact a connection has become established
in the course of evolution between pleasure and well-
being of the organism, pain and ill-being. The treatment
by Wohlgemuth in his article in the *British Journal of
Psychology* (Vol. 8, 1915–17), " Feelings, their neural
correlate and Pain," and his monograph, *Pleasure—
Unpleasure*, is avowedly incomplete. But we seem to be
justified in concluding that in general principle he would

[1] Perry, *General Theory of Value*, 284.
[2] *Zeitschrift für Psychologie*, Vol. 44 (1906–7), 1 ff. ; Vol. 75 (1916),
1 ff.
[3] Vol. 44, 29–30.
[4] Op. cit., 40.
[5] Op. cit., 15–16.

agree with Stumpf. For though he distinguishes pleasure
and unpleasure from sensations, yet he seems to regard
them as filling the same sort of function in mental life
as sensations, and as amenable to the same psychological
laws ; and he holds that they are connected with the
excitation of a feeling-centre in the brain. Others who
hold that a feeling-centre exists are Thalbitzer[1] and Head
and Holmes.[2] For all writers who take a view such as
this, there cannot, it would seem, logically be any question
of a necessary connection between feeling and action,
based on psychological grounds. If it is admitted that
such a connection exists, it can only be grounded on the
physiological fact that at a point in the " reflex arc ",
i.e. somewhere in the passage from stimulation of a sense
organ to motor discharge, a certain brain centre is usually
affected, the excitation of which is accompanied by the
conscious phenomena, which we know as pleasure and
unpleasure.

In the present work, it is proposed to present a version
of the theory, mentioned in the first place above, which
it is hoped may avoid some of the difficulties and contradictions hitherto felt to be involved in it. Inasmuch
as pleasure and unpleasure are held to be dependent on
the success of conation, our task, we shall find, will
carry us on to describe, as accurately as may be, the
nature of the main conations which run through both
the physical and mental life ; and thus we shall have to
discuss in some detail the nature of instinct. We shall
ultimately be led, it may be hoped, to form a more definite
idea of the whole mental life of man as a striving process.

A note should perhaps first be made on the question of
nomenclature. The generally recognised procedure now
is to use the word " pain " to denote a particular sort of
sensation derived from the skin or internal organs, and
the word " unpleasure " as the general term to denote the
feeling which is opposed to pleasure. This practice is

---

[1] *Emotion and Insanity*, 89–91.

[2] Brain, Vol. XXXIV, 1911, 102–254 ; see especially the conclusions,
180–2, and 190–2.

followed in this essay, though, as will doubtless be observed, it involves certain expressions which sound awkward and unusual to the ordinary reader. In particular the word " unpleasure " may appear to describe something which is a mere negation of pleasure, and to be inadequate to the more acute forms of suffering, in which the feeling certainly appears *primâ facie* to include a positive element, something more than a mere privation. Unless however a positive term can be found, which at the same time will not be confused with the bodily sensation of pain, there seems to be no choice but to follow the present practice in psychological writings. As a further point in nomenclature it may be observed that provisionally we shall use the word " feeling " as an equivalent for " pleasure and unpleasure." This course is convenient for the sake of brevity, and in accordance with the general view that pleasure and unpleasure are the only cases of " feeling ". We do not however wish necessarily to imply concurrence with this view. The question whether there are varieties of " feeling " other than pleasure or unpleasure is one which we shall have to refer to later.

PART II

SENSORY PLEASURE AND UNPLEASURE

CHAPTER I

THE QUESTION STATED

IT would seem that the theory of feeling, which we have described as that derived from the teaching of Butler, must start by admitting a *primâ facie* distinction between two classes of feeling. Firstly there are the pleasures and unpleasures which appear to arise directly from bodily conditions, such as the feeling excited by the scent of a rose or by a prick on the skin, by a warm bath, or by severe muscular fatigue. Secondly there are pleasures and unpleasures connected with such instinctive tendencies as ambition and self-assertion, gregariousness or love of society, curiosity or desire of knowledge. Thus Prof. McDougall states that " living beings are natively endowed with dispositions or tendencies to strive towards certain goals proper to the species,"[1] and that pleasure and unpleasure are bound up with the success or the thwarting of such strivings. This is true *primâ facie* of the main instinctive tendencies, such as those mentioned above ; and the theory which connects pleasure and unpleasure with the success of conation has based itself in the first place on these facts. It meets however with a difficulty when it attempts to explain on the same lines those feelings which appear to arise directly from bodily conditions. We propose to consider in the first place, this class of feeling, which for short may be termed " sensory ", dealing later with the pleasure and unpleasure connected with the main instinctive tendencies.

[1] *British Journal of Psychology,* Jan. 1927, 171, etc.

The unpleasantness of a prick on the skin or of a noisome smell, the pleasantness of a sweet taste or of the scent of a rose, all appear at first sight to arise as immediate accompaniments of the given sensations and to be not at all dependent on the success or non-success of a pre-existent conation. The difficulty has long been recognized by all those who treat psychology purely as an analysis of the facts of consciousness. Stout, in the concluding chapter of his *Analytic Psychology*, admits (and to some extent justifies) the failure of psychology to analyse the simple sensory feelings, and hands over the matter to physiology. The Herbartian school, as represented by Nahlowsky, admitted the distinction so far as to refuse the name of feelings (Gefühle) to what we have termed sensory feelings.[1] Sweet tastes or unpleasant odours are termed " Betonte Empfindungen ". Their " tone " is due to the fact that they work in either a furthering or inhibiting way on the functions of the nerves concerned, as well as on those of the central organs and those of the vegetative life. But in such sensations it is said the soul itself is not directly concerned, though they may give rise to feeling, in the proper sense of the term, by causing changes of mood in the soul. Feeling in the true sense is the result of the interplay of ideas present in the soul, inasmuch as the ideas are the forces working in the soul.

The question then arises whether psychologists, at least those of the general school referred to above, are bound to admit the existence of two orders of feelings, to which the same theory does not apply. McDougall, in his article referred to above, has endeavoured to bring the pleasures and unpleasures of sense under the terms of a " conational ", or as he terms it " hormic ", theory. Taking taste as an example he states that a sweet taste in itself (as a cognitive fact) promotes the conative impulse to consume the food which has been taken in the

---

[1] See Nahlowsky, *Das Gefühlsben* (1862), 29 and 30, as well as other passages.

mouth, and that the total process is then pleasant in so
far as the conative impulse is intensified and satisfied.
It seems to me that here there is an endeavour to obtain
more from psychological analysis than it can possibly
yield. The fact, so far as given in consciousness, seems
to be that the pleasure is given as an independent psychical
fact existing in its own right, and that a conation to maintain the total pleasant experience arises coincidently
with it. It is not possible from introspection to ascribe
priority to either the pleasure or the conation (as indeed
Prof. McDougall quotes from Stout). We have some
justification in cases of this sort in appealing to the
ordinary use of language, with which men have done their
best to describe their mental experiences. In a case of
an unexpected sweet taste or sweet perfume, (and, of
course, the unexpected pleasant experience is here the
crucial instance), the ordinary man has always said and
continues to say: "Contrary to my expectations I
found the taste or the scent " (or other sensation) " quite
pleasant, and so I continued to enjoy it as long as I could."
He would be puzzled and fail to recognize the description
if he was told that he really found the taste pleasant for
the sole reason that he wanted to have it. At least he
would say that the pleasantness arose independently of
his consciously wanting the experience. Similar considerations will apply to the examples which Prof.
McDougall gives of unpleasant sensations. A painful
prick or puncture of the skin does not appear as unpleasant
simply for the reason that we fail to withdraw from it in
time. It appears as unpleasant, if it lasts long enough to
be perceived as a pain sensation. I hardly think we know
of any instance in which a stimulation of pain nerves,
sufficiently intense to reach the point of unpleasure,
yet fails to be unpleasant, because of the speed with which
it is terminated by withdrawal. And certain odours
appear to us unpleasant if they last long enough for their
peculiar character to be recognized, however speedily
we may be able to get away from them. Nor is it easy

to follow Prof. McDougall in his view that the pleasurableness of single colours or tones is entirely due to the success with which they can be discriminated from their surroundings or background. It is no doubt true that every sensation is conditioned and affected by the relation in which it stands to other sensations. But no theory of cognition can possibly hold that the whole being of every perception is constituted by these relations.[1] So surely should it be also with the feelings that accompany perceptions. In paying tribute to the results of the " Form psychology " we must not push the doctrine of relativity too far. A general or diffused brightness seems to us ordinarily pleasurable in itself ; a diffused gloom unpleasant and depressing. Many of us have our " favourite colour ", which we are inclined to prefer as a rule in all the different surroundings in which it may be found, even though certain contexts and surroundings may sometimes be found which " kill " it. The less-developed minds, savages and children, are said to show such a general preference for the colours at the red end of the spectrum. It can hardly be said that this is due to the intellectual satisfaction of distinguishing these colours from their background. In regard to tones the pleasantness, if any, which accompanies a pure tone, free from overtones, is so slight that it is difficult to base any argument on it. In regard to harmony it has no doubt been held that the pleasure of a harmonious chord is due to the ease and completeness with which it can be grasped as a complex whole of relations.[2] But I should hardly think this theory has been generally accepted as proved. The pleasure of a harmonious chord does not appear to immediate introspection to be of the same nature as that involved in the understanding and mastery of a

---

[1] Alles in der Welt steht in Verhältnissen, besteht aber nicht daraus. Ward, *Psychological Principles*, 89, quoting Stumpf (Everything in the world stands in relations, but does not consist of them).

[2] Watt, *The Foundations of Music*.

complex pattern, i.e. the satisfaction of a purely intellectual impulse. It seems rather to include the "warmth" of a directly sensuous element. The same may be said of the unpleasure of a discord; it seems something different from the bafflement of an intellectual impulse.

CHAPTER II

THE question then is how we are to think of the connection between conation and the feelings that arise from bodily causes. We have argued that we cannot regard such feelings as conditioned by the conations of the conscious self. The purpose of the first portion of this work will be to enquire whether we may not find an analogue of conation in the sense organs and the body generally which may condition the appearance of bodily pleasure and unpleasure.

Let us look first at the facts which physiology has described under the word " tonus ". Thalbitzer has recently written as follows : " In the course of time it became clear not only that tonus is characteristic of muscle cells, but that all cells, so long as they are living, are functioning to some extent, and have a certain tonus ; living cells never stand still, but always show a certain degree of their specific function."[1] To which we may add the following from Verworn : " This important fact [i.e. that different varieties of stimuli produce in the same object wholly similar reactions] shows that in every form of living substance there must exist an extraordinary inclination toward a specific series of processes. This sequence is continually present in slight degree and finds its expression in the spontaneous vital phenomena, but the slightest stimuli of all kinds augment the discharge of the processes always in the same characteristic sequence for each specific variety of living substance, just as the nitroglycerine molecule can always be made to disintegrate into the same constituents by mechanical, gal-

[1] Thalbitzer, *Emotion and Insanity*, 116.

vanic, or thermal influences."[1] Verworn seems careful
here to exclude the appearance of any psychical implication in his use of the word "inclination". But it has often
been felt by others that this permanent state of activity
must, in certain organs, be held to include something in
the nature of a " striving " towards a further functioning.
In regard to the muscular system Bain long ago stated
this categorically in his theory of spontaneous movement.
" The muscles never undergo an entire relaxation during
life. Even in profound slumber they possess a certain
degree of tension or rigidity. This state is excited through
the medium of the nerves. The inference is that at all
times a stream of nervous energy flows to the muscles
irrespective of stimulation from without." " As the
battery of the torpedo becomes charged by the mere
course of nutrition and requires to be periodically relieved
by being poured upon some object or other, so we may
suppose that the jaws of the tiger, the fangs of the serpent,
the spinning apparatus of the spider, require at intervals
to have some objects to spend themselves upon."[2] In
regard to the sense organs Thalbitzer writes : " In order
that a sensation may arise there is need not only of a
stimulus, of an impression from the outside world, but also
of a certain activity, a movement towards the impression,
of a readiness for it, without which no sensation at all
can arise."[3] That this activity exists in the form of a
craving has been more definitely stated by Groos, and the
view is indeed fundamental to his whole theory of human
play. " Thus, as Jodl maintains in agreement with Beaunis
and others, every sensory tract not only possesses the
passive capacity of receiving and working up certain
stimuli, but also it presents itself from the first in the
form of desire for satisfaction with appropriate stimuli."[4]

It would seem as though in the unstimulated sense
organ (the appropriate brain centre of course included)

---

[1] Verworn, *General Physiology*, 474.
[2] Bain, *Mental and Moral Science*, 14 and 17 (shortened).
[3] Thalbitzer, op. cit., 27, cf. 122.
[4] Groos, *Spiele der Menschen* (1899), 5 (translated).

there must exist a state describable as tension, or *nisus*, towards the discharge of its peculiar function, a tension which will be increased, according to the state of nourishment of the organ, and the length of time during which it has remained unstimulated, within the limit at which atrophy through disuse may commence. If such tension has any effect on the main stream of consciousness, it will take the form of certain somewhat indefinite sensations in the organs concerned, accompanied by restlessness and an impulse towards their fuller activity. This impulse, by reason of its quality and localization, will not be entirely blind, but will naturally yield some awareness of the direction towards which it tends, though fuller knowledge of the end to be attained will be given in as far as there is memory of past satisfaction. It would be easily intelligible that this local restlessness or tension would, in general, not become focal for consciousness, but would fall into the general mass of the bodily sensations forming the constant background of the mental life. A mental factor, which is either constant or in process of gradual change, would naturally tend to be marginal for attention. On the other hand, the abrupt change that occurs when the craving of the sense organ is satisfied, would naturally force itself into the focus of attention and the feeling of satisfaction accompanying the change would be noticed, though the previous state of want had not been noticed. This explanation of the facts is as old as Plato. " Things which experience gradual withdrawings and emptyings of their nature and great and sudden replenishments, fail to perceive the emptying but are sensible of the replenishment, and so they occasion no pain but the greatest pleasure to the mortal part of the soul, as is manifest in the case of perfumes."[1]

If we examine the actual course of some unexpected

---

[1] *Timæus*, 65 (Jowett's Translation). The quotation is used in illustration of the view given above, though it must be admitted that Plato himself does not maintain it consistently. In the *Philebus* (51 and 52) he classes the pleasures of smell with the so-called pure pleasures, those which are not necessarily preceded by any craving.

pleasant experience, we shall I think find this view substantiated. Suppose that a pleasant sweet taste is
experienced, which has been preceded by no conscious
desire. The first moment of the sweet taste does seem to
occur as the satisfaction of a need. We can detect an
implied thought, which if put into words would run :
" This gives me something which I was just wanting."
The awakened craving is not as a rule satisfied by this
first moment, which appears as something incomplete.
The energy of the craving prolongs itself and seeks to
maintain and intensify the sensation, while the experience lasts, while the sweet, for example, is being dissolved
in the mouth. This continues until satiety is felt as attained, and this we must believe to be due to the fact
that the tension of the nervous elements concerned has
now been worked off and removed. During the process
thus described movements are often employed to intensify
the sensation, or reinstate it, as it appears to fade away ;
for example, shifting the position of the sweet in the
mouth. The process no doubt finds its natural end in the
act of swallowing. But this is because the sweet sensation acts also as a sign for the satisfaction of a further
impulse, one of the nature of hunger.

The existence of cravings in a subconscious form is,
as I think, further substantiated by the facts of desire.
It has always been difficult to see how from the mere
idea of a possible pleasant experience active desire should
be awakened, for in itself the idea of a pleasant experience
should itself be pleasant, and we should tend to rest in it
without effort towards change. Desire, so it has often
therefore been held, does not come into existence without
the *vis a tergo* of a pre-existent felt need, which, at least
if sufficiently intense, is unpleasantly toned. But on the
other hand it seems a fact of ordinary experience that the
suggestion of a pleasant sensation, say, the eating of a
sweet, provokes immediate desire, though no need was
felt beforehand. This difficulty appears to be satisfactorily solved by the theory that the want existed

c

previously in a subconscious form. When, after a state in which we are conscious of no desire for a sweet, the eating of a sweet is suggested, and becomes an object of desire, it seems to me that an actual craving is experienced in the sense organ ; and it seems natural to believe that what has happened has been the evocation of the need for stimulation from a subliminal stage and its intensification in consciousness. Primarily this stimulus-hunger would exist in the nerve endings of the tongue which mediate the sensation of sweetness ; but often also, no doubt, in the case we are using as an example, the physiological need of the organism as a whole for sugar might translate itself into consciousness as an element in the felt craving. We shall, however, deal further on a little more fully with the psychology of the " desire for pleasure ".

We may now endeavour to pass in review the main departments of sense in order to see what confirmation is obtainable of the general view thus stated. In regard to smell, which Plato used as his example in the quotation above, it is possible to say very little owing to the little that is known physiologically on the subject. No satisfactory classification has been made of the different olfactory sensations ; nor is it known whether there is any difference in the nerve endings which are active in different sorts of smell. It would seem highly probable, however, that the feelings going with the olfactory sensations are connected much more with the general organic effects than with the special form of the activity in the organ itself. Closely related as this sense has been in the past history of our mammalian ancestors with the nutritive functions and also to some extent with the reproductive functions, it would seem that a close connection between it and other bodily activities has been established, and that the feelings both of pleasure and unpleasure which occur with smells are the result mainly of these other bodily activities which they elicit. This is perhaps as much as we can say with regard to the reasons why one smell is pleasant and another unpleasant. We do, however, find that a certain craving for strong flavours does exist in connection with food. Flavourless foods appear insipid, and particularly amongst the less cultured there is a demand for such strong flavours as garlic with their food.

As regards taste we have already used sweetness as our example above.

The other main forms of taste sensation, salt, sour, and even bitter, are undoubtedly pleasant at low degrees of intensity as ingredients in dishes, and as affording variety they are liked. With increasing intensity they become soon unpleasant.[1] Külpe states that according to the experiments of Kiesow on tastes the course runs regularly from pleasure to unpleasure if the intensity of the stimulus increases.[2] It is, however, the special characteristic of taste sensations that they have a dual rôle. There is a pleasure due to the stimulation of the taste nerves themselves. And also, doubtless owing to connections established in racial history, these sensations act as excitants to the craving of hunger. Tasteless foods are usually uninteresting, and salt and other condiments are used to correct this.

It might be thought that the sensations given by the pain nerves afford an argument against the view taken here, being unpleasant at all degrees of intensity. It can, however, now be regarded as accepted that the slight stimulation of " pain spots " yields a sensation which is not unpleasant. The following description is given by Titchener.[3] " The sensation obtained from the pain spots then occurs in three stages : first as a bright, itchy sensation, secondly as prick or wiry thrill, and thirdly as punctiform pain." These sensations, at low intensities, are often noticeably pleasant. The stinging sensation of bay rum on the skin after a shave is distinctly gratifying.

[1] See, as regards sourness and bitterness, Wohlgemuth, *Pleasure—Unpleasure*, 25 (Expt. W. 27) ; 30 (Expt. W. 55) ; 83 (Expt. X. 81); 99 (Expt. X. 162); cf. p. 88 (Expt. X. 110), where the observer states that though a bitter taste was unpleasant, " in its extension it has something satisfying about it, due, I should say, to the faint stimulation of a number of end organs."

[2] Külpe, *Vorlesungen über Psychologie* (1920), 262 (though I have been unable to trace these experiments recorded).

[3] *Text Book of Psychology*, 152–3.

It is probably due to slight stimulation of pain nerves. So, too, are the burning sensations given by pepper and mustard, which, like a salt taste, are sought as remedies against insipidity. Children often seem to find injuries, apparently painful in character, rather interesting and exciting than unpleasant and seek to have them repeated.[1] Wohlgemuth in his experiments finds on a number of occasions that pain sensations of a slight character are adjudged to be pleasant by his observers.[2] Amongst these are the pricking and burning sensations given with the taste of acetic acid, and those yielded by a bristle prick or coarse sand-paper applied to the skin. In ordinary life, too, we are well acquainted with the pleasure often obtained by rubbing with a rough towel or hard brush and from scratching. Undoubtedly sensations from the pain nerves as well as tactual sensations form a part of these experiences. In the case of pain, as in that of certain tastes, we cannot explain why the point of overstimulation is reached apparently so much earlier in certain nerves than in others. It can only be taken as a fact in the physiological make-up of the organism that the nerves mediating sweet taste, for example, are able to endure stronger stimulation than those mediating bitter tastes. For an explanation, if such exists, we should probably be driven back to the facts of racial history.

It must also be admitted that very rarely if ever are we conscious of any craving for stimulation of the pain nerves, comparable in any degree to the craving, say, for a sweet taste. This, however, need not appear strange. We may perhaps assume it as a physiological fact that the energy of discharge in the well-nourished organism drains towards certain organs in the body rather than towards others, and that normally there exists little activity of tension in the unstimulated pain nerves. When, however, the pleasantness of such stimulation has

---

[1] Shinn, *Notes on Development of a Child*, I, 149–51. Sully, *Studies of Childhood*, 221–2.

[2] Wohlgemuth in *British Journal of Psychology*, Vol. 8 (1915–17), 450 ; *Pleasure—Unpleasure*, 165 and 217.

been once experienced, there does arise a desire for repetition ; and on our view this can only be interpreted as the coming to consciousness of a pre-existent tension or craving.

The pleasures connected with the temperature senses are very largely due to secondary organic effects. Thus the result of a warm bath is to open and cleanse the pores, so that the healthy action of the skin is promoted, and also to induce a dilatation of the blood vessels at the periphery, so that circulation is made more rapid, the tissues, etc., receive a richer alimentation, and the general nutritive changes are speeded up. At the same time, however, we cannot doubt that here, too, the satisfaction of a craving for stimulation also plays a part. In our climate the temperature of the air is nearly always below that of the body, and the end-organs for warmth are stimulated far less than those for cold. Hence, when at intervals, for instance by a warm bath in cool or cold weather, they receive due stimulation, this will naturally give rise to a pleasure of its own. A further source of the pleasure in a warm bath, we may add, is probably the gentle, almost " caressing ", stimulation which the cutaneous nerves of touch receive from the surrounding water.[1] It is doubtless the coincidence of these satisfactions from various sources which goes to make up the very high degree of physical pleasure which we experience in a warm bath.

In passing to the other senses more directly concerned with cognition the same principles may be found to apply, though under somewhat different conditions. These senses, especially sight and hearing, are in our ordinary life constantly in receipt of stimulation ; and it might be thought that the impulse to discharge their specific functions might be thus continuously satisfied. Similar cravings are, however, to be found if we look at the facts in more detail, especially at the earlier stages of life. It is well established that one of the first facts observed in

---

[1] This is remarked by Groos, *Spiele der Menschen*, p. 15.

the new-born infant is a " general expression and behaviour of contentment in mild light, and sometimes of
discontent at its withdrawal ".[1] Very soon, as early as the
third week, according to Miss Shinn, there are observed
movements which tend to bring recurrence of the gaze
to favourite spots (bright patches of colour and illuminated
surfaces). Miss Shinn believes these to be conditioned by
a craving of the sensory cells for light stimulus.[2] " There
seems to be from the first in the developing sense cells not
merely the capacity of receiving stimulus, but an actual
craving for it, a tension and discomfort in its absence
which stimulates motor reaction. There is thus a movement, a ranging to and fro of the eye, which is thus steadily
directed by the pleasure feeling, at first automatically,
and then by an easy development becomes voluntary
movement, determined by association with pleasant
experiences."[3]

It is thus highly probable that the craving of the eye
for light stimulus is the most important factor in the early
part of the process of development by which the child
learns to perceive and know its external world. But
whether or no we follow Miss Shinn in her detailed account
of the process, there can be no doubt of the pleasure
given in early life by the mere exercise of sight. " The
pleasure in the exercise of vision at this stage is reported
over and over by all observers—demonstrations of joy
in glitter, in strong chiaroscuro, in moving and vibrating
objects, and in the human face with its changing high
lights."[4] In the early development of knowledge of the
external world by touch sensations, it is possible to hold
that the same principle plays an equally important part.
" The original touch-organ of the suckling is not the hand
but the mouth."[5] The persistent carrying of objects to
the mouth which takes place in the first year of childhood
cannot be explained by the desire to eat. " The mouth ",

[1] Shinn, op. cit., II, 22.   [2] Shinn, op. cit., II, 53–4.
[3] Shinn, op. cit., II, 58.   [4] Shinn, op. cit., II, 62.
[5] Koffka, *Growth of the Mind*, 251.

says Stern,[1] "performs the task of explaining and confirming, by its more familiar and exact touch sensations, the new and indistinct impressions of the other organs (hand and eye) ". And Miss Shinn explains the facts in the same way as for the development of visual perception. " The whole behaviour of the infant in the early months shows that the mouth does crave touch and muscular sensation, as the eye craves light ; the highly charged cells of its sensory centres are in continual state of tension, which demands discharge by the appropriate stimulus."[2] It is impossible here to go into the development in detail. But according to Miss Shinn it is from the craving to have and reinstate touch sensations that the child is led on towards the most important part of its intellectual development, the correlation of sight and touch sensations. No doubt other accounts of the cognitive development of the child are given ; but as far as I can see, unless the explanation given in Miss Shinn's work is adopted, no other can be given except in the form of the automatic maturation of nervous connections and compounding of reflexes, explanations which are in the last resort of the mechanical type.

In our ordinary life no doubt we are not conscious of any need for the stimulation of the senses mainly concerned in the cognition of the external world, sight, hearing, and touch. In the statement of one of the observers in Wohlgemuth's experiments on feeling, however, there occurs what seems an interesting exemplification of a view, similar to that here put forward, in regard to a craving for tactual sensation. The stimulus consisted in the particular case of the skin being rubbed with velvet first very lightly and then more heavily. Here is the observer's introspective report : " The first slightly unpleasant. The sensation consisted partly of slight tickling and partly of very light successive contact sensations, producing altogether an impulse to withdraw the hand.

[1] *Psychology of Early Childhood,* 115.
[2] Op. cit., II, 86, cf. the summary of development given on pp. 96–7.

An attitude of dissatisfaction towards it as something inadequate. The second slightly agreeable, less tickling,
a more satisfying series of contact sensations, the attitude
changing to one of comparative satisfaction at its
adequacy. There is observable a kind of appetite in the
skin for gentle stimulation, so that more of it can be more
gratifying (a wish to go on)."[1] I think observation does
confirm that this sort of attitude is not uncommon in
ordinary life. A very slight stimulus (in other spheres of
sense as well as in touch) does appear as inadequate and
evokes an appetite for a stronger and more satisfying
stimulation.

In the spheres of sight and hearing a craving of this
character does undoubtedly become conscious, if, when
the organism is well nourished and not fatigued, there is
abnormal deprivation of the appropriate stimuli. In
such circumstances complete darkness and silence are
felt as irritating and " oppressive ". We should be tensely
watching and listening for something ; and the occurrence
of a stimulus would be felt as a pleasant relief. Intense
glare of light and unusually loud noises are on the other
hand very unpleasant, and so is unduly prolonged stimulation with the same kind of light or sound, which leads to
unpleasant sensations of fatigue. Thus we are naturally
led to the conclusion that there is a certain optimal
degree of stimulation for which the nerves of these organs
crave and in which a feeling of pleasure is experienced,
and that beyond this degree unpleasure arises.[2]

In Grant Allen's work *Physiological Æsthetics* an
attempt has been made to explain the sensory foundations
of beauty on these lines. He points out that in nature
the colours at the red end of the spectrum are much less
common than those at the violet end ; and thus the rarer
stimulants of reds and yellows are the more distinctly
pleasurable in themselves as arousing function in seldom-

---

[1] Wohlgemuth, *Pleasure—Unpleasure*, 78, Expt. X, 52.
[2] This is not unlike the view of Herbert Spencer, *Principles of
Psychology*, I, 273–7.

excited nerves.[1] At least, this is undoubtedly the case
for short periods and with minds of primitive type, and
with children, while with the civilized adult it is probable
that associations play so large a part in the appreciation
of colour, that the natural and exclusive effect of colour
stimulus is obscured. The colours at the red end of the
spectrum, in fact, have a greater thermal value than those
at the violet end. From the psychological point of view
they may be described as more stimulating and exciting,
yielding a coarser and more violent form of sensation than
the " cold " colours ; all of which explains the preference
which is shown for them by primitive and unsophisticated
minds. That such a mind finds great pleasure in glitter
and bright colour need hardly be insisted on. The value
placed on such precious stones as sapphire, ruby, and
emerald must have had its origin in a delight in pure
colour. Grant Allen goes further and attempts to explain
the pleasurableness of colour combinations on the same
lines.[2] He starts with the fact that combinations of the
complementary colours, e.g. blue and yellow, green and
red, are as a rule very pleasing. This is due to the fact
that the nervous apparatus employed in the seeing of red
(for example) is assumed to have suffered some sort of
fatigue ; in a green sensation, then, fresh and unused
nervous tracts are excited, and this affords the apparatus
involved in red a measure of rest and recuperation.
The pleasure is due to the fact that the demand for exercise on the part of unused nervous tracts is met. This
interpretation was supported by the explanation given
of the complementary after-sensation. After fixation of
a red surface, the apparatus involved is fatigued, and when
the eye is stimulated with ordinary white light only those
rays in the white light which excite a green sensation are
able to produce an effect. In this explanation Grant
Allen took for granted Helmholtz's theory of colour vision.
This is, of course, matter of considerable doubt. In
particular the view that the complementary after-

[1] *Physiological Æsthetics*, 154.   [2] Op. cit., 161 *et seq.*

sensation is any sort of fatigue-phenomenon is usually considered to be disproved. But if we turn to Hering's theory of colour vision, it is, I think, possible to base on it a similar theory of the pleasurableness of colour contrasts. According to Hering yellow (for example) causes a katabolic, or dissimilation, change in the yellow-blue apparatus, and blue an anabolic (or assimilation) change in the same apparatus. After stimulation with either of these colours, the apparatus in question tends to return to equilibrium by developing the process opposite to that which has just occurred; the complementary colour thus being automatically evoked, and affording the basis for the complementary after-sensation. By stimulation with (say) blue light the anabolism which has occurred has resulted in the formation of a large quantity of " material ". If stimulation by yellow light now occurs, the normal katabolic or " breaking-down " process will be increased owing to the amount of material available, and the resulting sensation will be intensified, and the process of return to equilibrium assisted. That this should mean an increase of pleasantness will be fully in accord with the theory we are now outlining. For intensification of a normal process (not reaching the point of overstimulation) must mean an increased activity of nervous tracts which will satisfy more completely their inherent need of stimulation.

This need of a more completely satisfying stimulation of the sense organs is not usually felt by the ordinary person, no doubt. But in some who have developed a special sensitivity it is probably a constant factor; the sensitive artist finds it difficult to put up with the ugly and harsh sights of our great cities and prefers as a rule to live in surroundings where the nerves are more harmoniously stimulated.

If we turn to the sphere of sound, it must be admitted that at present no physiological theory of the nature of harmony exists, which is even plausible. We have given reasons above for holding that an explanation on a purely intellectual basis does not seem satisfactory. One must believe that a basis for harmony may yet be found in some form of sensory "synergy", as Stumpf thought to be probable, though he could formulate no definite theory.[1]

The theory which we have endeavoured to sketch and illustrate as above would thus regard sensory pleasure as dependent on the need of stimulation inherent in the sensory nerves. So far as our knowledge of the sense organs goes, it would seem that there is an adequate degree of stimulation of each organ at which the resulting sensation appears as pleasant ; while the course, which any experience of unexpected pleasure runs, follows the same lines as given in the case of a sweet taste. At the first phase there is evoked a conation in the form of a conscious craving, which directs itself to the maintenance of the sensation until the total experience is worked out to its normal conclusion in satiety.

I would maintain that this theory is on the whole substantiated by the facts reviewed. But there are further questions to be settled before the account can be regarded as in any way complete. The question that meets us now is whether we are to regard the state of want or craving as essentially unpleasant, and whether, if so, the pleasure of satisfaction consists solely in (or is conditional on) the removal of the previous unpleasure, or whether, and in what form, pleasure is to be regarded as a positive element in the mental life. This is the point with which Plato and Aristotle were largely concerned in their treatment of the subject ; and the distinction drawn above is expressed in the discussion whether pleasure is the accompaniment of ἀναπλήρωσις (replenishment or restoration) or of ἐνέργεια (vital activity), which is an end in itself. The endeavour to state the opinions of the Greek philosophers on this matter in a consistent form would hardly be in place here. A good description of the theories of pleasure held by different philosophers is given from this point of view in Sir W.

[1] Stumpf, *Ton Psychologie*, II, 214.

Hamilton's *Lectures on Metaphysics*,[1] and is brought down
as far as Kant. Kant may be taken as typical of those
who hold that the occurrence of pleasure is entirely
conditional on the previous occurrence of pain or unpleasure. " Pleasure is the feeling of the furtherance of
life, pain of its obstruction. . . . Therefore every pleasure
must be preceded by pain ; pain is always the first.
For what would follow on a continued advancement of
vital force, which indeed cannot be heightened beyond
a certain degree, except a speedy death from joy ? Moreover no pleasure can follow immediately on another ;
but between the one and the other pain must intervene.
It is the slight depressions of vital power, with intervening
expansions of it, which make up the state of health, and
which we erroneously take for a continuously felt state
of well-being, whereas it really only consists of pleasant
feelings following each other intermittently, i.e. always
with pain occurring in between. Pain is the stimulus
of activity and in activity we first become conscious of
life ; without pain a lifeless state would ensue."[2] In
so far as this is held to apply to the whole of the mental
life, and not only to the bodily sensations, we shall hope
to deal further with it later on. At present we are concerned only with the bodily life ; and on taking a somewhat nearer view of this, I hardly think ordinary experience is found to bear out the Kantian view. The first
point we have to observe is this, that even though the
preceding craving may have been fully conscious, yet
the intensity of the pleasure which is felt when sensory
nerves are stimulated after rest, is in many cases quite
out of proportion to the intensity of the craving. The
satisfaction is certainly in such cases a good deal more
than merely the removal of the unpleasure of the craving.
The pleasure seems to us to consist in the fact that im-

---

[1] Lecture 43 (Vol. II, 444 *et seq.*).
[2] Kant, *Anthropologie in pragmatischer Hinsicht*, § 60. It is, I
suppose, the case that these views, which are applied by Kant to all
the mental life, and not only to the bodily sensations, had some influence
on the better-known pessimism of Schopenhauer.

pulses or tendencies, possessing a positive value of their own, which had been obstructed, are now given free play. The normal process of the physical life consists partly in processes which are relatively constant and unchanged, such as respiration, circulation, and glandular secretions, and partly in processes which demand a certain rhythmic alternation of want and satisfaction over relatively long periods, such as nutrition and digestion, muscular exercise and repose, and so on. The processes of the first class do affect consciousness in some degree, according as they are subject to slight accidental variations; and thus their condition goes to make up the general sensation of bodily life. But in general they have very little effect on consciousness unless there is some abrupt interference with them. We must always, however, be to some extent conscious of the processes of the second class. I think we see, on looking at them, in regard to feeling, that they do not consist in alternations of pleasure and unpleasure, which balance one another. The case is rather this. The total alternating process of want and satisfaction, if it proceeds within certain normal limits, is felt as slightly tinged with pleasure. A felt need or craving, if it remains within a moderate limit, or if it moves continuously towards satisfaction, is not as such unpleasant. It only becomes unpleasant if the tension involved in it increases beyond a certain limit, owing to delay in satisfaction or the absence of any progress towards satisfaction. Take the case of hunger. A condition of moderate hunger does not usually appear to us unpleasant; but rather as adding a sort of " zest " to life, and the existence of this feeling does not appear to be dependent necessarily on any clearly present idea of coming satisfaction. Frequently we do not observe it at all until eating actually begins, or food is perceived either by sight or smell. It only becomes definitely unpleasant if there is undue delay in satisfaction, in which case the gnawing pains of hunger (due to the contractions of the empty stomach) become intense enough to be painful and are accompanied by general sensations of bodily weakness or deficiency.

Muscular exercise may be taken as another example and may be considered somewhat more fully. The free exercise of limbs and muscles, when we are fresh and vigorous, may be extremely exhilarating and pleasurable. The beneficial effects of exercise are described physiologically as follows : " The speeding up of the metabolic activity of the body, which is a characteristic feature of exercise, involves the more rapid utilisation of reserve nutritive material and probably also the more complete oxidation of these materials within the cells. In this way it prevents the cells from being clogged with substances awaiting combustion or with waste products awaiting removal, and enables the lamp of life to burn more brightly."[1] This accounts for the greater part of the pleasurableness of muscular exercise, though we must allow that " stimulus-hunger " plays a certain rôle here also. Well-nourished and unexercised muscles are in a state of tension and restlessness, the reflection of which in consciousness is due to the message sent to the sensory centres of the muscular sense. This state of tension finds its natural outlet in the discharge of muscular energy, towards which it directly points. But muscular exercise can be highly pleasant without a pre-existing stage in which either the relative stagnation of the inactive bodily system, or the restless tension of the unexercised muscles, appears as definitely unpleasant. No doubt confinement, in which the free use of limbs is prevented, is a highly unpleasant state : and after such confinement the free exercise of the body is rendered the more pleasant, but there is no need for such a stage to have pre-existed.

It is not entirely certain to what physiological conditions the sensation of fatigue is due. The conclusions given by Bainbridge[2] are very largely negative. In

---

[1] Bainbridge, *Physiology of Muscular Exercise*, 184.
[2] *Physiology of Muscular Exercise*, 176–80.

general terms it is, however, probable that there result from muscular work various products of metabolism, that these at a certain stage of exertion accumulate in the blood and tissues to an extent sufficient to interfere with the working of the nervous and muscular system which is being employed, and that such products at the same time affect the sensory nerve endings in the muscles, joints, and tendons so as to give rise to the sensations of fatigue. Under the driving force of some instinctive impulse or some conscious purpose derived from a higher mental stratum, work is often continued after fatigue has reached a considerable degree of intensity, and nerves and muscles affected by the fatigue conditions are thus called on to function beyond the capacity which they possess at the time. The more extreme forms of this experience are very unpleasant. But, it seems to me, there is often a period in the concluding stages of muscular exercise when a "healthy tiredness" is felt which is not unpleasant. There is a feeling bound up with the consciousness of having worked out for the time being the capacity for exercise of the organs concerned, of having satisfied a natural craving of the organism ; it is a state in which an instinctive urge appears to have reached its term. It is highly probable that the physiological conditions of fatigue have begun at this stage, for it is hardly possible that the craving for exercise should be worked out at the exact moment before these conditions begin in any form, however slight. Thus slight sensations of fatigue may be held to be not unpleasant ; but may appear as a normal stage in the working out of a natural process. No clearly held ideas are necessary as to what constitutes a healthy bodily life ; nothing more than a feeling going with the fact of the normal alternating processes of healthy exist-ence. It is, however, probable that in such incipient fatigue there is a decrease of the pleasure felt in muscular exercise ; and this decrease of pleasure may be felt as a hint or warning of future unpleasure in its positive form. After this state of moderate fatigue rest and reparation then appear as the normal continuation of the alternating process. After fatiguing work which has reached the stage of unpleasantness, rest is extremely pleasant. It is difficult to regard this as having any other source than the processes of reparation in the nervous tissue which has been fatigued, i.e. the gradual re-establishment in it of the normal metabolism. " The pleasures of repose correspond both in their general diffusion and in their specific localisation to the pains of fatigue. After holding out a weight with the arm till the exertion has become painful, the relief which follows discontinuance of the action is both general and special. We have a conspicuous pleasure which we refer directly to the cessation of muscular exertion in the arm ; and we also have a vaguely localised satisfaction in resting the whole body and in sitting or lying down."[1] To the same causes also no doubt we are justified in attributing the feelings going with rest after moderate fatigue which has not been unpleasant.[2]

We may also glance at the case of the sexual function. The pleasureableness of the sexual acts appears to depend on a high activity of discharge taking place in certain glands, which only function to the full extent at relatively long intervals. There often occurs, no doubt, a certain

---

[1] Stout, *Analytic Psychology*, II, 297–8.

[2] There are some authors who, regarding pleasure as essentially bound up with the exercise or activity of the nervous system, fail, as it seems to me, to take sufficient account of the pleasure of repose. The already quoted theory of Lehmann (see p. 3) suffers, it seems to me, from two defects. In the first place, it seems most probable that there are stages of exercise, after rest and nourishment, in which dissimilation exceeds assimilation, and yet the exercise is pleasurable. In the second place, it is obvious that there are many periods of bodily life in which assimilation exceeds dissimilation. Lehmann has not stated anywhere in his work what he holds to be the result for sensation and feeling during such periods. But it seems impossible to doubt that the " building up " processes in the nervous system after exhaustion are accompanied by sensation. If there is consciousness of fatigue, there must be consciousness also of the passing away of fatigue.

According to Marshall (*Pain, Pleasure and Æsthetics*, 204 and 324) pleasure occurs whenever the stimulus affecting an organ occasions the use of surplus-stored force. In order to account for the pleasure of repose he has to suppose it to be due entirely to the release of activity in other organs of the body which had been quiescent while the fatigued organs were active (pp. 209–213). This supposition is criticized by Stout (*Analytic Psychology*, II, 296–7).

bodily restlessness, amounting to unpleasure, if the sexual impulse is denied its normal exercise. But it must be obvious that in sexual acts there is a high degree of pleasure, which has a positive quality of its own, and is not dependent on, or indeed as regards degree, related in any way to, such a state of pre-existing tension or craving.

As regards the special senses it is obvious from our preceding discussion that the craving for stimulation does not necessarily mean unpleasure. Such craving, as long as it is not too intense, repeatedly remains in the subconscious level ; and even when it rises to be clearly conscious, it is not definitely unpleasant, as long as stimulation is not unduly withheld.

Thus we may see, I think, that in most of the main functions of the bodily life there is a certain periodicity or rhythmic alternation of want and satisfaction, and that the total process may, if going on normally, be tinged with a feeling which we may describe as " goodness " or " worth-whileness ". It is indeed the very fact of the alternation that gives us the chief part of our feeling of life. I believe that ordinary introspection does bear this out, and that there is justification for the common opinion that in normal health there is this, usually slight, feeling of " goodness " attaching to the bodily life, though the proviso should be added incidentally that for the most part this must remain in the background of the conscious mental life, and that to make the bodily life the constant object of attention tends rather to destroy its pleasantness and to conduce to states of anxiety. We should not be understood, of course, to assert that the pleasantness of the normal bodily life always remains at the same level. It is plain that at the time when those organs whose actions are intermittent and crave stimulation receive the due amount of stimulation, there is a heightened feeling of pleasure, doubtless the result of a heightened bodily activity. On the other hand, at the periods of want, say even a moderate hunger, there is a lower degree of bodily activity and of pleasantness. Undoubtedly

D

there is a certain difference between the occasions of pleasant feeling corresponding to that drawn by the Greeks between ἀναπλήρωσις and ἐνέργεια; but in our view this is a difference of degree and not of kind. When, say, after a period of abnormal confinement and gloom, ordinary slight exercise and fresh air are felt as pleasurable, this is the result of the sudden change from a depressed state of the vital functions to one of increased activity, though this is not of the degree which would under other circumstances be felt as pleasurable. But when from a normal bodily condition we pass to some exhilarating exercise, skating or tobogganing, for example, the pleasure felt is equally the result of a speeding up of the vital function. The difference is that in the one case the start is made, as it were, from a lower level of vital activity than in the other. In this respect most of the pleasures of the special senses, especially those of sight and hearing, must be held to belong to the latter class. They are related to an enhancement of function which has not as a rule been preceded by any marked depression. In each sort of case there is, or may be, consciously experienced an inner urge towards the increased activity, and psychically this certainly seems somewhat different according as the present state is positively unpleasant or not. The difference consists in this, that, where unpleasure is felt, the impulse takes the form in consciousness of a movement *away from* the present state, whereas otherwise the turning away from the present is less emphasized in consciousness, and it is rather the future state *towards* which movement is made, which is important for consciousness. This however does not appear as an ultimate difference of kind. Undoubtedly the inner " urge " or conation towards alteration of the existing state becomes especially prominent in the former case, and this must be due to the fact that the current of the physical life has been as it were dammed, with a resulting increase of the energy of the impulse towards normal function. At such times there is either actual unpleasure, or at least a lowered degree of pleasantness, which is able to act as a hint or warning of the possibility of unpleasure to come in the future. It would seem that there goes with the bodily processes, of which we have spoken, a psychical accompaniment in the form of an effort or conation to maintain them in their normal course, but that this conative factor does not tend to come into the conscious centre of the mental life, unless there is felt a certain degree of depression or obstruction of the vital processes, in which case there is conscious effort to restore them. This does not apply only to states of deprivation such as hunger. The beginning of over-stimulation may also be interpreted by the mind as a sign of possible future unpleasure, for example, incipient fatigue in muscular exercise, or satiety in eating. Thus the course of the normal bodily life as experienced seems to present itself as a series of self-maintaining processes, tinged throughout with a slightly pleasurable feeling, which may become strong when stimulation is received after a period of intermission, and guarded against any undue excess in the direction either of overstrain or of deficiency by feeling, which being less pleasant, points in the direction of unpleasure and acts as a sign of possible future disturbance or depression of vital activity. We may also therefore assume that those bodily processes which are constant and not periodic are similarly self-maintaining in character. For, though when proceeding normally they may add little or nothing to the conscious mental life, we know that as soon as they are obstructed, acute conscious unpleasure may arise, with effort to terminate the impeded conditions and restore the normal course of life. A certain confirmation of this view of the affective character of the bodily life may, I think, be found in the case of those patients, who have lost an important part of those organic sensations, which go to constitute the general sense of life. Sollier writes as follows of persons with a high degree of visceral anæsthesia—" Psychically there is loss of memory, sometimes enormous aprosexia, apathy, and indifference to

everything, both things and persons, complete absence
of appetite and also of all desire, all need, except that for
an automatic perambulation up to the day when the
strength is inadequate for it. . . . With these subjects
then an inhibition of the visceral functions is sufficient
to let us see the appearance of a state of indifference, of
moral anæsthesia, and of extreme lack of emotivity,
while the general sensibility and the special senses are
affected only a little or not at all, any more than the power
of movement and the muscular sense."[1] Plainly the loss
of the visceral sensations means that the bodily life is
lived without zest, on one dull and apathetic level, and
this loss of affective tone may extend to the mental life
generally (though we are not concerned here with the
question of the loss of emotion generally). Normally,
however, it would follow that the healthy bodily life, with
its periodic rhythm of need and satisfaction, is carried on
with a pleasurable zest, slight but quite able to be detected;
and I think our ordinary observation of ourselves will
tend to confirm this. We cannot enter here fully on the
general question whether neutral states of consciousness
exist, a question which has often been discussed. But
we can point to certain authors who have held that pleasure is the accompaniment of all normal bodily sensations.
Bradley has written as follows : " Let us say, pleasure
is the feeling which goes with presentation when that has
not got the conditions of pain. A sensation is pleasant
when not psychically or physiologically discordant.
Pleasure thus will be the result of such positive conditions
as imply the absence of pain. It will be the attendant
either of *all* normal sensations, or of merely those where its
(unknown) conditions of quantity or quality are present."[2]
Grant Allen's theory may also be quoted : " Pleasure is
the concomitant of the healthy action of any or all of the
organs or members supplied with afferent cerebro-spinal
nerves, to an extent not exceeding the ordinary powers of

---

[1] Sollier, *Le Mécanisme des Emotions*, 153 (translated).
[2] Bradley, *Pleasure, Pain, Desire and Volition, Mind*, No. 49 (1888), 7.

reparation possessed by the system."[1]   And he adds further on : " Doubtless every activity when not excessive, nor of a sort to prove destructive to the tissues, is in itself faintly pleasurable : indeed, we generally recognise this fact in our ordinary language ; but owing to the commonness and faintness of the feeling, we habitually disregard it."[2]

---

[1] Grant Allen, *Physiological Æsthetics*, 21.   [2] Op. cit., 24.

CHAPTER III

THE THEORY OF SENSORY UNPLEASURE

ARE we then to say simply that pleasure is the feeling which accompanies the normal exercise or enhancement of some or all of the vital functions, and unpleasure is the feeling which goes with the opposite condition, i.e. with their depression ? This is obviously true in a general way and in accordance with the general assumptions on which human conduct as a rule is based. Many apparent exceptions, such as poisons harmful though pleasant, and medicines, beneficial though unpleasant, can be explained without difficulty on the basis of the distinction between local stimulus and diffused effect. It is quite possible for a drug to stimulate the nerves of taste to a degree of activity which is pleasant, while at the same time a gradual depression of vitality is being brought about in the body generally.

If, however, it is sought to give the theory thus stated the status of a scientific law, it soon becomes apparent that difficulties arise. Starting in the 'eighties of last century, numerous attempts have been made, largely by experiment in psychological laboratories, to discover what, if any, are the constant bodily manifestations of the psychical states of pleasure and unpleasure. The object has been, it may be presumed, mainly to test the invariable truth of the coincidence between pleasure and vitality, unpleasure and the reverse. It is usually considered that these experiments have led to no reliable results. The facts to which observation has mainly been directed have been those connected with respiration, action of the heart, circulation, and the force exercised by the voluntary muscles.

A certain number of those observers who claim to obtain definite results have affirmed that in states of pleasure breathing is shallower and quicker, while the pulse becomes stronger and slower ; while in unpleasure the results are reversed, a deeper and slower respiration and a quicker and weaker pulse.[1] On the other hand, a number of other investigators deny that either the respiration or the pulse show any uniform change corresponding to the existence of pleasurable and unpleasurable feelings in the mind ;[2] they assert in general that such changes as take place are correlated rather with the intensity of the affective condition or emotion involved and the general state of excitement and activity than with the presence of agreeable or disagreeable feeling.[3] All these results are obtained with the comparatively weak stimuli, which, at least in the case of unpleasure, are all that is possible to employ in these laboratory experiments. Mantegazza,[4] observing the effect on the heart in the case of bodily torture sufficient to cause severe suffering inflicted on animals, found that " pain diminished the frequency of heartbeats in the rabbit, rat, and chicken, and the diminution measured with great exactness the degree of the pain " ; and that a severe pain of ten minutes may have a depressing effect on the heart's action lasting several hours. It is well known that in severe pain suffered by human beings the action of the heart usually becomes irregular, or it may sometimes be temporarily inhibited. Though it is obvious that in acute unpleasure, associated as it is as a rule with some abnormal bodily state, there is disturbance of the heart's action as of other bodily processes, yet it is not always easy to interpret the effects

[1] Wundt, *Philosophische Studien*, Vol. 15 (1899), 163. Zoneff and Meumann, *Philosophische Studien*, Vol. 18 (1903), 57. Alechseiff, *Psychologische Studien* (1907), 156 ff.
[2] Angell and Thompson, *Psychological Review* (1899), Vol. 6, 32 ff. Shepard, *American Journal of Psychology*, Vol. 17 (1906), 522 ff.
[3] E.g. Angell and Thompson, op. cit., 41.
[4] *Physiologie de la douleur* (1888) (French translation), 39 and 40. Mantegazza apparently inflicted severe pains on animals with a view to observing the results. Probably this is the only time this is likely to be done.

as phenomena of depression. Wundt, regarding acceleration of the pulse as the regular accompaniment of unpleasure, states that it is due to a removal of the regulatory
effect which the Vagus normally exercises on the heart,
and thus may be the result of an inhibiting effect on the
Vagus centre in the brain ; acceleration of the pulse thus
being the result of a lowered activity in the brain.[1]
While all the facts are not easy to interpret, it would
undoubtedly be the general view that in acute unpleasure
the phenomena of the heart's action are those of depression or at least disorganisation.

It has been often claimed that changes in the circulation have been found corresponding regularly to the state
of pleasure or unpleasure. A pleasant stimulus has been
said to cause vaso-dilatation in the limbs, bringing about
a rise of volume, sometimes preceded by an initial fall,
while unpleasant stimuli cause a simple fall in volume.
Similar changes are said sometimes also to occur in the
brain, i.e. vaso-dilatation in pleasure, and vaso-constriction
in unpleasure.[2] If these facts could be established, they
would be of theoretical importance ; for an increased
circulation would mean a livelier metabolism in the
tissues, and therewith a general raising of the vital
powers and the capacity for work ; while the opposite
results would ensue on the obstructed circulation going
with vaso-constriction. They are, however, disputed by
other investigators. Angell and Thompson[3] state that
almost all their emotional experiences, whether agreeable
or disagreeable, produced vaso-constriction. Shepard[4]
finds that all moderate nervous activity, whether pleasant
or unpleasant, tends to constrict the peripheral vessels,
and to increase the volume and size of pulse in the brain.
The volume of the hand often rises a little before the

[1] *Physiologische Psychologie*, 6th ed., II, 371 and 372.
[2] Myers, *Experimental Psychology*, 309. Lehmann, *Die körperlichen Aeusserungen psychischer Zustände*, Part I, 116 and 136 ; Part III, 489. Previous conclusions in the same sense had been reached by Meynert, Lange, Féré, and others.
[3] *Psychological Review* (1899), Vol. 6, 53.
[4] *American Journal of Psychology*, Vol. 17, 1906, 558.

decrease sets in ; the volume of the brain increases at first, then falls to normal, and then increases again.[1] This is in accordance with the results of Mosso,[2] the originator of experiments on the volume of the limbs, who found that in any emotion, even when a person is merely spoken to and awakened from a drowsy indifferent condition, there is contraction of the blood-vessels in the extremities and flow of blood to the brain. Cannon[3] states that at times of pain and excitement blood is driven from the abdominal viscera into the central nervous system, i.e. the lungs, heart, and the active skeletal muscles, this being an adaptive function rendering the body more fit to meet a struggle or other emergency. It is moreover patent that the results as regards circulation phenomena will be complicated with those regarding the action of the heart, and on the whole it does not seem that there are results connecting vaso-constriction or vaso-dilatation in any simple way with conscious pleasure and unpleasure.

Experiments to test the power of the voluntary or skeletal muscles have been of two sorts. In the first place a pleasant or unpleasant stimulus is inflicted on the subject, who, immediately after, is instructed to pull with his maximum force on the dynamometer ; the result is recorded and compared with those obtained in the absence of the stimulus. Secondly, the subject is instructed to grasp the dynamometer as forcibly as possible, a pleasant or unpleasant stimulus is then exhibited to him and the result on the pre-existing contraction is recorded and compared with that obtained in the absence of a stimulus. Féré, who originated experiments of the first class, declared the result to be that in general every peripheral excitation causes an increase of potential energy, and a strong excitation affecting sight, hearing, smell or taste, causes with normal subjects an increase

[1] Loc. cit., 544-5.
[2] Mosso, Fear (1896), 100 ; also 82 and passim.
[3] Cannon, Bodily Changes in Pain, Hunger, Fear and Rage (1920), 106-9 and 200-2, and vide Behan, Pain, etc., 120-1.

in the force exercised.[1] But, he goes on to say, unpleasant excitation constitutes an exception, stimulation in itself is pleasant (as Aristotle said at the opening of the Metaphysics), but unpleasant sensations, involving as they do overstrain of the organs concerned, result in a decrease of the energy shown by muscular contractions.[2] There can be little doubt that Féré's results can be accepted as regards the general effect of stimulation. Any excitation at one point of the organism, as long as it is not exhausting, does seem to determine a diffused wave of energy which spreads over the rest of the organism, and seeks discharge. Mosso gives the following example which is interesting.[3] A colleague (Fabrizi) whose normal power was represented by a pressure of 4·35 kilogram meters, testing himself at a period of considerable mental excitement just before delivery of his first lecture, found his power raised to the figure of 5·95. It is, however, more than doubtful whether Féré was right in saying that unpleasant stimuli cause a decrease in muscular energy. Some of his own figures raise the doubt. Thus with a subject whose normal pressure on the dynamometer was represented by the figure 23, Féré found that under stimulation with red light the figure was 42, with orange 35, with yellow 30, with green 28, with blue 24 ; and he connects these figures with the greater pleasantness of the colours at the red end of the spectrum.[4] But for the same subject he gives the following results as regards stimulation with tastes : sugar 29, salt 35, sulphate of quinine 39, figures which show the stimulating effect on muscular contraction varying inversely with the pleasantness.[5] Mainly with the object of testing Féré's conclusions further detailed experiments were carried out by Störring and Rose. Störring[6] found that there was nearly always a decided increase of the motor effect through unpleasure, as compared with that in the state of indifference. He could find little, if any,

[1] *Sensation et Mouvement*, 51, and 32.   [2] Op. cit., 62–6.
[3] Mosso, *Fatigue* (1906), 257.
[4] Féré, op. cit., 42 and 62.   [5] Op. cit., 47.
[6] *Archiv für ges. Psych.*, Vol. 6 (1906), 347–55.

increase of the motor effect in states of pleasure ; and in
any case the effect was less than under conditions of
unpleasure. Rose[1], whose experiments seem more detailed and thorough than any of the preceding, declares
that in most cases unpleasure causes an increase of the
strength of the reaction as compared with the indifference
state ; and the greater the degree of the unpleasure, the
less variable is this result. He draws a distinction between two of his subjects, classed as active-minded, and
the rest. The former declared that they were conscious
of the unpleasure as giving a motor impulse, either
because the movement distracted from the unpleasure,
or because of a general feeling of excitement.[2] The other
five denied that the unpleasure consciously influenced
the motor impulse.[3] But it is interesting to note that
in their case the strength of the reaction increased proportionately as much as that of the " active-minded "
(although the quickness of reaction increased somewhat
less). Rose apparently did not experiment with pleasant
stimuli. It would seem, however, as though we are
justified from these experiments in concluding that in
states of unpleasure there is a tendency, for the most part
automatic or involuntary, towards a nervous excitement
which finds an outlet in strong muscular contraction. If
we turn to experiments of the second class we find results
which seem at first to be contradictory of the above. It
is stated that the effect of pleasant or unpleasant stimuli
on already contracted muscles is as follows : " A very
pleasant stimulus usually causes an initial drop followed
by a significant rise in the tracing ; after which the tracing
gradually falls, though maintaining a higher level than
usual. A very unpleasant stimulus causes a decided fall
in the tracing, after which there is a gradual fall, the
tracing maintaining a lower level than usual."[4] In the
absence of stimulation when the subject tries to maintain

[1] *Archiv. für ges. Psych.*, Vol. 28 (1913), 149–52 and 166, fig. 4.
[2] Op. cit., 111–13.   [3] Op. cit., 113–15.
[4] Myers, *Experimental Psychology*, 311.

a state of maximal contraction the result is an obliquely descending almost unbroken line. Lehmann gives a similar statement of the result which unpleasurable feeling causes on muscular work consisting of a series of rapid pulls instead of a constant contraction.[1] But he explains that this is due to the existence of conscious factors in the process. The maintenance of the pre-existing task demands a certain concentration of the attention. Any stimulus, whether pleasant or unpleasant, causes an initial distraction of the attention, but such distraction is greater and more continuous in the case of unpleasure than of pleasure. Thus we may readily believe that in the case of unpleasure the distraction of the attention has more effect than any automatic increase of innervation could have. In the case of pleasure the higher level of the tracing subsequently maintained may be due to the excitatory effect of the pleasant stimulus, which Féré also believed that he found. Moreover, when unpleasure occurs during the performance of a certain task, the agent would probably feel some half-conscious tendency to associate the action and the unpleasure. The further impulse would be then not to maintain the existing action or movement, but to alter it. The movement caused by an unpleasant experience will tend in a certain direction, that towards removal of the stimulus, whereas the movements resulting from pleasant experience are diffused and exuberant, the expression of an increase of general vital energy. That the above result of unpleasant experience should spring from clearly conscious purpose it does not seem necessary to suppose. Thus we are not called on to admit that these results of the effect of unpleasure on previously existing contraction contradict those derived from the effect of unpleasure on new movement.

The defect of all these experiments carried out in psychological laboratories is that they can only make use as a rule of weak stimuli (especially in the case of un-

[1] *Die Hauptgesetze des menschlichen Gefühlslebens*, 299.

pleasure) which have a transient effect. Mantegazza's experiments on animals have been already referred to above in regard to the action of the heart. He also found that injuries adequate to cause severe pain brought about a notable diminution of the bodily temperature ; while if there were violent muscular contractions (i.e. struggles) the fall, though less, still existed ; the fall often lasted long after the pain had ceased.[1] He further states that the carbonic acid exhaled diminishes as a rule very considerably ; but when there is violent movement the action of the pain is counteracted by the influence of movement, and the final result may be a very large increase in the carbonic acid exhaled.[2] It would seem that these results point to a certain conflict in the case of animals between the phenomena of vital depression on the one hand and the tendencies to reaction and activity on the other. It is quite possible that in the case of animals the phenomena of depression due to bodily injury may appear sometimes more simply than in the case of men, and less complicated by active nervous reaction, and that where there was little reaction, there was little actual unpleasure experienced.

There are permanent states of unpleasure (melancholia) in which we seem to find the phenomena of vital depression in a more easily observed form than is the case with unpleasant experiences, due to momentary stimuli, the effects of which are transient. G. Dumas states that the vital functions generally are depressed in all cases of melancholia, whether the melancholia be (in his terminology) of active or passive nature. There is loss of weight as compared with the normal, reduction of the functions of organic combustion, as shown by the amount of urea excreted and carbonic acid exhaled, and lowered tempperature.[3] Where there is active melancholy there is generally less reduction in these functions, but they are still below the normal. In speaking of active melancholy he means to refer to those cases in which there is acute

[1] *Physiologie de la Douleur*, 30, 31.   [2] Op. cit., 57–61.
[3] *La Tristesse et la Joie*, 280, 291, 295, 307 ff.

mental suffering. Always, he says, where in melancholiacs we meet signs of activity in pulse, muscular
movement, secretion and ideation, there we shall also
meet mental pain.[1] There is far more suffering in active
melancholy than in passive. And he considers that the
probability is that the two forms of melancholy (active
and passive) correspond to the two results following on
any shock which deranges the nervous system. Sometimes
the shock paralyses ; in other cases it provokes violent
reactions and cries ; and which happens doubtless depends
on the original sensibility of the subject.[2] Throughout he
treats the amount of suffering as bound up with, and
varying with, the amount of resistance offered to an
injury or shock, originally mental in character but tending
to cause a general vital depression. There are certain
other cases which might be quoted as disproving the correlation of vital depression, in itself, with unpleasure.
Külpe cites from Mignard a description of certain patients,
who he denotes Béats, with whom are found much the
same phenomena of physical depression as amongst
the passive melancholiacs, but who mentally are per-
fectly content with everything, avoid all exertion and
remain sunk in happy repose. The difference according
to Mignard is that passive melancholy involves a state of
felt inhibition, in which the subject feels himself impeded
from being as he would, whereas "" Béatitude " is the
sluggard's existence, the running down of all bodily
conditions, which demands no exertion and is left to itself.[3]
Thus we may conclude that no degree of melancholy is
likely to be felt at all, unless there is resistance and struggle
against the conditions, at least to some extent.

That the capacity to feel bodily pain is in itself a sign
of a certain amount of vitality, is a fact that is universally
recognized. Narcotics or anæsthetics are drugs which
have the power completely to paralyse and abolish the
action of the nerves concerned, and if administered in

---

[1] Op. cit., 29.   [2] Op. cit., 110.
[3] Külpe, *Vorlesungen über Psychologie* (1920), 276–7.

sufficiently large quantities they bring about a painless death. We do not, of course, find the abolition of feeling without that of sensation as well. But if the depression were in itself unpleasant, the gradual approach of unconsciousness, the gradual raising of the threshold, for the sensation in any nervous tract, should be accompanied by some form of physical unpleasure. Lehmann has drawn attention to the fact that if after one of the larger intestinal operations the patient feels himself particularly light and well, it is almost certainly the sign of a fatal termination ; but when the sick person complains of internal pain, it is a sign of healing and favourable progress. The absence of pain must doubtless be taken as a sign that the internal organs have perished and so become insensible.[1] We may also here mention the well-known " euphoria " of the dying, which seems to occur when the organism has ceased to struggle against disease, and life is ebbing away. In the same way is doubtless to be explained what sometimes may have seemed a singular contradiction in the life of the organism, namely that excessive heat stimulation, i.e. scorching and burning, is accompanied by intense unpleasure, whereas excessive cold stimulation, though in the form of frostbite it may be equally fatal, is frequently accompanied by no feeling at all. The fact would appear to be that though cold as a stimulus acts on certain cutaneous nerve organs, yet, as Verworn states, it is only increase of temperature that must as a rule be regarded as a stimulus which effects an excitation in living substance. " Those stimuli which depend on the diminution of vital conditions, e.g. decrease of the surrounding temperature, appear in general with increasing intensity to depress vital phenomena without previous excitation."[2] It is true that in certain cases absence of the normal stimulus does cause a degree of acute unpleasure, not merely the unpleasure of craving, in living beings, for instance the acute suffering of asphyxia

[1] Lehmann, *Die Hauptgesetze des menschlichen Gefühlslebens*, 242.
[2] Verworn, *General Physiology*, 470.

or the pains of hunger. In both these cases, however, the acute suffering must probably be considered as the result of some over-stimulation which occurs as a secondary result of the absence of the normal stimulus. In asphyxia, due to deprivation of oxygen, acute unpleasure and convulsive struggles occur. They are the result of the toxic action of unoxygenated blood on the respiratory centre in the medulla. The " gnawing pains " of hunger have been shown to be due to the violent contractions of the empty stomach and other parts of the alimentary canal.[1] It is not known by what agency these contractions are brought about ; but it is possible that they may be due to the presence of some toxic product in the empty intestines.[2]

As a last piece of evidence on the point before us, we may adduce the conclusions of Cannon as to bodily changes in pain and great emotional excitement. This investigator has shown that in such conditions there occur in the body changes which, while partially unfavourable from the vegetative point of view, yet are favourable as adapting the body for great temporary exertion. These changes include the temporary inhibition of digestive activity[3], diversion of blood supply from the abdominal regions to the heart, lungs, brain and limbs[4], and increase of sugar in the blood.[5] They all tend to occur in any case in emotional excitement, but an important agent in either initiating or increasing them is the increase of secretion from the adrenal glands into the blood.

We should not, of course, be understood to imply from the foregoing that the capacity of feeling unpleasure is always proportionate to the vitality of the organism. There are states of fatigue, or other abnormal states, in which the threshold of unpleasure feeling is lowered below the normal. There is a condition of weakness in which

---

[1] Cannon, *Bodily Changes in Pain, Hunger, Fear and Rage*, chap. XIII.
[2] See on this point, Cannon, op. cit., 261.
[3] Cannon, op. cit., 19.   [4] Cannon, op. cit., 106–9.
[5] Cannon, op. cit., 66–79.

the living substance of the organism is abnormally unstable and liable to discharge. These must be considered as states in which a small amount of excitation results in exhaustion, owing to the unduly low reserve store possessed by the organism.[1] But it remains true that there is more vitality in these conditions than in one of analgesia.

The evidence thus cited above is no doubt hardly sufficient to enable us to form a definite picture of the bodily processes which occur in feeling. It does, however, enable us to see that in certain cases at least bodily unpleasure is a phenomenon, not simply of depressed vitality, but of such depression complicated with reaction and struggle against it in the organism. Such cases are in general those of a stimulation, due to outside action, which is excessive relative to the capacity of the organism as a whole or that of some particular organ. It has been stated as a general rule by Verworn that, with increasing intensity of stimulus, excitation, in the form of increased activity of dissimilatory processes, is first increased, and then at a certain point gives way to depression ; which if the stimulation is still continued, may lead to paralysis and death.[2] If any conclusions are to be drawn as regards psychical accompaniments, it seems at least highly improbable that an activity would cease to be pleasant, as long as it continues without any damage to, or exhaustion of, the nerves concerned ; and thus unpleasure would commence at or about the point of time at which the stimulation is beginning to have its depressing effect. A mere depression, however, in one part of the organism could not by itself result in increased activity elsewhere. There must be some place at which the increased activity shown in unpleasure commences ; and on our theory this could only be in the affected organ, which continues in some degree to function against, or in spite of, the tendency to depression. If, therefore, the net result of an initial

---

[1] See this explanation given by Lehmann, *Die Hauptgesetze des menschlichen Gefühlslebens*, 244.

[2] Verworn, *General Physiology*, 470. Cf. 396 for effects of heat, and 428 for effects of electrical and chemical stimuli.

depression is an ultimate increase of activity, we seem entitled to regard the energy shown as having the form of a reaction or struggle against the depression.

We can regard this reaction as occurring automatically, in the first place, as an organic phenomenon. The effect on the main stream of consciousness will depend on more than one factor—in the first place, on the intensity of the process involved as compared with that of the processes taking place in the other parts of the psycho-physical system at the same time, and the consequent direction of the attention. An abrupt change of considerable magnitude will, of course, force itself on the attention at once. Small injuries or impediments to vital processes may not be noticed for some time, or their resulting sensations may form part of the undistinguished mass of the bodily sensations, if attention is concentrated in some other direction. But at a later moment of less concentrated attention, hitherto unnoticed bodily sensations will probably affect the main stream of consciousnesss, and amongst them the pain due to the pre-existing injury, and therewith will occur a feeling of unpleasure and conscious aversion. Or to take another example, a mark or sign of abrasion may be seen on the skin, and this may suggest the idea of pain. A sensation previously unnoticed will thus be strengthened, and we may become conscious that a slight sensation of pain " has been there all the time ". The aversion felt at once in all these cases derives in our view directly from the already given effort of the organism to function against, or in spite of, the injury. While the bodily sensations appertain essentially to the objective .side of conscious experience, yet the existence of the conscious self is immediately bound up, in a way not to be further analysed or accounted for, with their maintenance in a certain form, that is to say, with the maintenance of the normal bodily life. As soon as conscious unpleasure arises, there occurs therewith an attitude of the self in which it rejects the disturbance, and, as it were, sides with the effort towards normal bodily functioning. This attitude is an integral part of the total experience of conscious unpleasure and cannot be separated from it. We must distinguish this primary aversion from ideas of an abstract character derived from memory, which may add themselves to it at a slightly later stage, as, for example, the idea that a bodily injury, if unhealed, may prejudice health and activity in the future.

In the second place, the effect on consciousness may depend on how far the organism is able to provide an automatic remedy. We know that there exist in the body protective arrangements, which function automatically and quite without consciousness, so as to get rid of obstructions and restore the normal course of the bodily process. There are other cases in which obstructions are got rid of in a way which appears partly automatic and partly voluntary. When a small foreign body lodges in the larynx there takes place that act of quick inspiration and abrupt expiration which we call " coughing " and which may succeed in ejecting the intruding substance. This act is accompanied by consciousness. But usually it takes place automatically without being consciously purposed, sometimes it can be carried out intentionally, and it is also possible as a rule to prevent its occurrence by conscious effort. Lastly, there are cases in which no pre-existing mechanism works automatically to get rid of an obstructing body, and varied voluntary movements, different in each case, have to be carried out ; if, for example, a thorn is lodged in the skin. We obtain, I would suggest, a consistent view of all these phenomena if we regard them as illustrating different stages of automatization through heredity. The basis in each case must be regarded as the effort of the affected organ to function in spite of some obstacle which tends to obstruct or depress its normal working. The first result of this reaction will be varied effort and struggle, which will continue if possible until the obstruction is removed. In the course of evolution various protective mechanisms have grown up, which work immediately and automatically and therefore have tended to lose all psychical accompaniment. According as no such hereditary mechanism exists, it still remains necessary for the organism to seek with varied effort to restore the normal course of its life ; and in such cases we find in consciousness actual feelings of unpleasure, together with the conation to terminate the condition of unpleasure. Wundt[1] and others, as is well known, have held that all the presently existing automatic mechanisms of the body represent purposive movements, which have degenerated into automatism through constant repetition. There is no need for us here to go so far as to argue this question. It is enough to point out that the " expelling " or " getting rid of " reflexes, of which we here speak, may be regarded as having a special position. They are not an essential part of the functions of the organs concerned. Their origin must have occurred *after* the organ has been, in some degree at least, established in its working functions, inasmuch as they are protective arrangements, safeguarding those functions. It seems therefore a highly probable supposition that what has happened has been that the living body, reacting with varied effort against obstruction, has had to make use of and adapt as far as possible its pre-existing structure in order to re-establish the normal course of its functions. It may be admitted that in the foregoing there is a good deal of purely hypothetical construction. At the same time, it may be claimed that from the point of view of " economy " there is an advantage in endeavouring to view the phenomena called vital and those called psychical from a single standpoint.

It may be worth while to add that in speaking of a reaction by the organism we are not asserting the existence of any new source of energy. Doubtless the resources available for the reaction are limited by the energy already

---

[1] Chief passages in Wundt are, I think, *Physiologische Psychologie*, III, 247–52, and *System der Philosophie*, I, 324–5. We may cf. Koffka, *Growth of the Mind*, 108.

stored in the organism. We have been concerned with the *form* which the output of energy takes. On the other hand, there is no need to conclude that the net result of the reaction to an unpleasant stimulus is always more exhausting to the whole organism than would have been the case without such reaction. This has been often asserted, e.g. by Bain, Ribot, Féré, Dumas.[1] But the net result of an active response to an unpleasant stimulus, if only of moderate intensity, may be an increase of vital energy as compared with a condition of stagnation or non-response. We know in ordinary experience that the result of pain is often stimulating.

We have however now also to admit the existence of other cases in which the behaviour of the organism in regard to over-stimulation is different to that just described. When action of an organ continues for too long a time, fatigue occurs, due, as previously stated in regard to muscular exercise, to the production of waste products which lower the capacity for work. Physiology appears to be doubtful whether fatigue is also due to the over-consumption of substances that are necessary to activity, i.e. to the fact of waste of tissue outrunning repair ; but it seems probable that this must be the case in cases where nervous elements only are concerned, e.g. the continuous excitation of the retina, leading to fatigue of the eye. In any case, in the state of fatigue the capacity of the organ for work is lowered. As a consequence of the fact that work is impeded there is naturally a tendency for work to cease. If cessation of action takes place at once, or at any rate before the difficulty of continuing work has reached more than a moderate stage, unpleasure will not occur. But often under the influence of a dominant idea derived from a higher mental stratum, or as the result of instinct, habit, or perhaps mere inertia, work goes on for some time after fatigue has reached a fairly

---

[1] Bain, *Senses and Intellect*, 309 and 310. Ribot, *Psychology of the Emotions*, 30. Féré, *Sensation et Mouvement*, 65 and 130. Dumas, *La Tristesse et la Joie*, 351.

acute stage. The conscious self in the early stages of this process will be engaged on the side of continuing activity, and the fatigue conditions will be regarded as a hindrance to it. But sooner or later the impulse to cease work must prevail, if the complete destruction of the organ is to be avoided, and therefore the impulse to stop will become the will of the conscious self. The condition we have just described may be general, as well as local. There is the condition of general tiredness or sleepiness, the exact physiological cause of which appears to be doubtful, but is probably some sort of fatigue state of the central nervous system. Sleep involves a general suspension or lowering of those bodily activities with which consciousness especially is connected, i.e. those of the higher nervous centres with the sensory organs and the voluntary muscles subordinate to them, while only the vegetative functions continue normally. In the state of sleepiness, which is a tendency towards sleep, noises or other forms of sensory stimulation are unpleasant, but the unpleasantness does not appear to have the same local character as that due to the continued stimulation of some fatigued organ. We feel the unpleasure rather as due to the fact that our progress towards sleep is interrupted. The fact that lies behind this unpleasure must be a discord or struggle between the tendencies created by the sensation and those of the sleep impulse. Every incoming sensation brings about in the mind an impulse towards further activity with it, generally speaking in the direction of placing it in relation to other sensations. Thus it is a necessary preliminary to sleep to close the eyes, because visual sensations are constant when the eyes are open, and we are impelled to constant mental action in defining and ordering them. An intermittent noise is more disturbing to sleep than a constant one, because it calls up the active expectation of the next sound. The low sound of human conversation often disturbs us more than a louder meaningless noise, because we feel impelled towards trying to understand it. In all these cases of conflict, however, it is against the incoming stimulus that resentment is, or may be, felt, this showing that in the given moment the conscious mind is siding rather with the tendency towards lowering of the bodily activity than with that towards its enhancement. It is true, of course, that we cannot will the coming of sleep in the same way as we can will results directly within our power, such as either the production of bodily movement, or the retention or recall of ideas. Such effort to will sleep, with a conscious idea of its beneficial effects, involves a mental activity, which is usually self-defeating. But, partly by arranging external circumstances in a favourable way, we can let ourselves passively go in the direction of sleep, and the fact that the interruptions are resented does show that at the moment this is the predominant tendency of the mental life. We have to admit this as a fact in which life involves a certain self-contradiction. The higher nervous centres cannot energize continuously and at intervals require relaxation to a lower level of activity, involving either complete unconsciousness or an approximation to it. This periodical tendency is reflected in the felt mental impulse towards the lower level of consciousness, an impulse which must be called conative, but which must be held to be a contradiction of the essential nature of the will towards life. In it there prevails for the time at least that tendency against which conscious life is essentially a struggle. The close relationship, from the psychological point of view, between sleep and death has often been felt. It is described with force, even if the words may strike ordinary common sense as slightly exaggerated, by Sir T. Browne (in the *Religio Medici*). " 'Tis indeed a part of life that best expresseth death ; for every man truly lives so long as he acts his nature or some way makes good the faculties of himself. . . . It is that death by which we may be literally said to die daily ; a death which Adam died before his mortality ; a death whereby we live a middle and moderating point between life and death—in fine, so like death, I dare not trust it without my prayers and a half adieu to the world and take my farewell in a colloquy with God." It is possible to go further than this and to regard the contest between the will to life and the will to death as the underlying fact of all life. Thus Jung has written as follows :[1] " In the morning of life man painfully tears himself loose from his mother, from the domestic hearth, to rise through battle to the heights. Not seeing his worst enemy in front of him but bearing him within himself as a deadly longing for the depths within, for drowning in his own source, for becoming absorbed in the mother, his life is a constant struggle with death, a violent and transitory delivery from the always lurking night. This death is no external enemy, but a deep personal longing for quiet and for the profound peace of non-existence, for a dreamless sleep in the ebb and flow of the sea of life." There is truth, as well as force, in this statement no doubt ; but on looking into the matter I do not think that we should be justified in speaking of a will to death as though it were a " willing " on the same level with that to life. Looked at from the biological and physiological point of view the death of the higher organisms, in so far as it occurs from immanent causes, is not the result of action by the organism as a whole, but the result of the separate and independent action of parts of it, which assert their own impulses and destroy the co-ordination of the whole. In so far as such an organism acts as a whole, it must act for the preservation of the whole. The two terms are in fact synonymous as regards living beings. Weissmann, as is well known, held that life did not inevitably and necessarily tend towards its own dissolution and that unicellular organisms may be in fact immortal, in so far as they are not destroyed by some external agency. However that may be, at least it cannot be asserted as a self-evident fact, that death is the necessary obverse of the life process. From the psychological point of view,

[1] *Psychology of the Unconscious* (Wandlungen und Symbole der Libido), 390.

too, it seems difficult to speak of a " will to death ". Cases occur, of course, exceptionally, in which men destroy their own lives deliberately. But here we must consider the mental state to be rather one of intense aversion to the present condition of conscious existence than active desire for unconsciousness. Every desire must be given a content by some idea possessing a positive character of its own. Thus the so-called wish for non-existence must have as its content the present state of existence which is to be negated ; for the nothingness which is sought can only be defined as a negation of something now existing. Suicide does seem in point of fact to be inspired by intense aversion to the present, accompanied by only a wholly vague and indefinite idea of the future state, if any, which is to be substituted for it. But these cases are, if we consider the total number of mankind, extremely rare. For the ordinary human being, it is true to say that in proportion as he is alive and vigorous, his active willing is directed towards exercise of function, accompanied by a high degree of consciousness. At times there occurs a weariness leading to acquiescence in a state of lowered consciousness and in progress towards unconsciousness, which comes automatically through the action of the body, without being actively sought. In some cases this may be the chronic state of mind towards the end of life. There is a weariness of life which leads to acquiescence in the coming of death. Stevenson, it is true, writes :

> " Glad did I live and gladly die,
> And I laid me down with a will."

But I cannot help thinking that this is something of a distorted picture of the way in which the end of life is normally faced. I would suggest that the considerations we have given in the foregoing will be consistently completed if we regard life in a fashion somewhat similar to that in the metaphysics of Bergson. Life, according to this view, is the tendency to accumulate energy and to expend it in a high form of activity, as against the tendency of matter which is towards the levelling down of energy and a lower form of activity. " It is like an effort to raise a weight which falls."[1] " Life as a whole, from the initial impulsion which thrust it into the world, will appear as a wave which rises and is opposed by the descending movement of matter."[2] We can be content here to leave the dualism implied in these statements unresolved and need not follow Bergson in his attempt to find the origin of matter itself in a reversal of the original movement of the vital impulse. Life implies both the co-ordination into a unitary whole of the energies of the subordinate parts of matter which it uses and also a heightened degree of activity; and the result is increase in the level of consciousness; for as Bergson has said, life and consciousness are co-extensive.[3] That these two factors go together in the fact of life, we may see from our own conscious experience. Our moments of acutest consciousness are those when we act most as a unitary whole, concentrated towards some definite purpose, and not only subordinating to this all the bodily powers, but also making the largest possible use of the results of our past experience. On the other hand, the more distracted and dissipated is attention, the more each tendency in the organism is left to have its own way, for example, in the automatic play of the association of images or ideas, uncontrolled by purpose, the lower is the level of consciousness. Sleep must be considered as an extreme form of this; for in sleep there is a shutting off, for the time being, of the higher nervous centres from the sense organs and from the vegetative life, which continues to function more or less independently, while the higher centres, if they function at all, do so in a dissociated and independent manner, resulting in dreams. The vital impulse then, this tendency to increased co-ordination and heightened activity, seems to be engaged

[1] Bergson, *Creative Evolution*, 260.
[2] Op. cit., 284.   [3] Op. cit., 196.

in a constant struggle with the tendency to degradation and dissipation of energy belonging to the matter which it uses. In so far as life is preserved, that struggle is, of course, successful. The occasions which we have reviewed in the foregoing are those in which in various ways the struggle, of which the organism is the seat, reaches with some abruptness a point of intensity at which it becomes an acute discord ; and it is this situation which is reflected psychically in the feeling of unpleasure.

CHAPTER IV

LET us then endeavour to apply the results of the fore-going speculations in an attempted formulation of the nature of sensory pleasure and unpleasure.

Pleasure is the mental element which accompanies the sensations of the bodily processes when they proceed in a normal fashion. Ordinarily when they proceed smoothly without abrupt change, the pleasure being constant and slight is not observed and remains in the background of consciousness. When, as the result of a special stimulus, or for other reason, the normal process in the body or in any organ is, with a certain suddenness, raised to a higher degree of activity, in which, however, the limit is not overpassed, at which excessive waste or consumption of material begins, then the feeling of slight goodness which accompanies the normal process is raised to a higher degree ; and we have the feeling of pleasure in the acutely conscious form. Usually, when the stimulus acts on a special organ, the pleasant feeling will have its focus in that organ, where the activity originates, and there it will tend to be primarily localized. But the increased action of a single organ will always tend to have a reverberation of increased activity over the organism generally ; and this activity will itself be accompanied by pleasant feeling, which will appear as part of the total pleasant experience. Unpleasure is the mental element occurring as the result of the conflict between the vital impulse, that towards exercise and enhancement of the vital activities, and tendencies towards depression and stoppage of vital functions, whenever that conflict reaches a certain share of acuteness. There are two sorts of cause for this condition, under-stimulation and over-stimulation. (1) It is a case of under-stimulation when some external factor, on which vital activity depends, is absent or present in inadequate amount, e.g. warmth, food, or the kind of stimulus on which the several special senses depend for their excitation. Those organs which depend for their activity on external stimulus, are when unstimulated in a condition of lowered activity. According as they still possess a store of energy, there is present in them still an effort to function, which results in a state of slight tension. This condition is not in itself unpleasant and moreover, while the tension remains slight, the sensation will only form an indistinguished element in the mass of the bodily sensations. If, however, stimulus is withheld for an unduly long period, there will result an increasing tendency to depression and at the same time an increase also of the impulse to function and the tension, with the result that a positive feeling of unpleasure will appear in consciousness. When after such state of tension the required stimulation occurs, the activity of the organ will be the greater according to the intensity of the pre-existing tension and the store of energy available and will be accompanied by a proportionate degree of pleasure. (2) Over-stimulation has two forms, (a) over-action of some part of the body as the result of purely internal causes, (b) over-stimulation directly or indirectly due to the action of an external force. In the case of (a), the fatigued state of the organs in itself, involving as it does a diminished capacity for work, creates an impediment to further activity, and unpleasure is due to the fact of effort to function continuing against the resistance. As regards (b), which includes most of the acute bodily pains ordinarily so-called, the condition is probably the somewhat abrupt increase of dissimilatory over assimilatory processes in the nerves concerned, which proceeds beyond the point at which there is easy repair of the waste, and begins to lower the capacity of the nerves for reaction. If this tendency proceeded far enough, it would result in the complete paralysis or death of the nerves affected. But in the initial stages there occurs an automatic reaction against the tendency to depression and an effort still to function, on the part of the nerves, with such store of energy as they still possess. It is this state of discord that is felt as acute physical unpleasure. Unpleasure, whether resulting from under- or over-stimulation, will as a rule tend to be local ised in that part of the nervous system primarily affected. But there will always also be a tendency towards a reverberation over the organism generally. The diffused effects would seem to be of the same nature as the process in the local organ, i.e. a conflict between the tendencies to activity and those to depression of the vital functions.

Our view is thus that bodily pleasure and unpleasure depend on an analogue of conation existing in the organism, a *nisus* to maintain, or to carry out to the full extent, the functions proper to the bodily system. They are the results for consciousness of a process of the nature of conation, which has taken place in the nervous system, without the direct co-operation of the conscious self; pleasure being the feeling of the success and smooth working of that process, and unpleasure of its obstructed working.

But in order to complete our account of the psychological facts it is necessary to define somewhat further the course of the affective phenomena which results. It follows from the foregoing that with every sensory pleasure or unpleasure there is inseparably bound up an act of primary acceptance or rejection. It is what we ordinarily term " like " and " dislike ". Ordinary language and thought assume these to be part of the feelings in question. To be " pleased " is the same thing as to like and accept, at least momentarily; to be " displeased " the same as to dislike and reject. In the case of the sensory feelings we hold that what is present here is nothing but the emergence into consciousness of the conation already present in the organism. The primary liking and acceptance of the pleasant experience is constituted by the effort towards a more complete functioning on the part of the nervous elements concerned, which continues its energy into the period of satisfaction, and the results of which have become for the moment focal for consciousness. The primary dislike and rejection of the unpleasant experience in the case of fatigue, represents simply the fact that there is a tendency towards stoppage of the activity and that this tendency is beginning to prevail over the impulse to action ; and in the case of over-stimulation by external agency it is nothing but the direct outcome of the automatic nervous reaction against the depression tendency, when continued into consciousness in the manner which we have already described.

To these primary acts there adds itself normally a further conative and affective series. In the case of pleasure this in general has no very marked character. The impulse in pleasure is to let things take their own course. As long as the pleasant experience lasts, it will tend to maintain itself with a certain energy, which is prepared at any moment to resist interruption. Movement will only be called for in so far as it is necessary in order to maintain the pleasant sensation and prevent its slipping away. A conscious feeling of general contentment may accompany the experience. As regards unpleasure, when an activity ceases as the result of fatigue, no further affective results follow. In the case of acute unpleasure due to external stimulation the results in conation and emotion are more striking. McDougall[1] states as a result of his own introspection that any sudden pain sensation excites a momentary fear, though it may often be so faint and fleeting as to be hardly recognisable. He treats this fear as the conative response automatically evoked by the sensation, i.e. by the cognitive fact. I feel inclined to agree that a note of fear is the usual consequence of sudden pain sensation, if at all acute. But that it invariably goes with pain sensation as

[1] *British Journal of Psychology*, Jan. 1927, 176.

such, may appear doubtful. Nor is pain the only unpleasant sensation which excites fear. The slightest hint
of asphyxia tends to provoke an immediate fear, and so
often does the " sinking " sensation in acute hunger, or
indeed the sensation of any severe organic disturbance.
Moreover, on McDougall's theory it is difficult to see how
he would avoid being compelled to regard the emotion of
fear as the accompaniment, in itself unnecessary and
meaningless, of a withdrawal impulse which would
ultimately be of a mechanical or " tropistic " character.
The following is, I would suggest, the general course
which these events follow. The process of the bodily
life is, as we have said, a self-maintaining one ; it tends to
prolong itself into the future with a certain " momentum ", which has a conative character. The consciousness
which goes with the bodily process is normally accompanied by an affective factor, a slight pleasantness, which
is in general in the background of the mental life. If an
abrupt change occurs involving a sudden depression of,
or impediment to, the vital processes, then as we have said
there may occur the feeling of acute unpleasure, when
there is a reaction by the nervous elements concerned
against the depression tendency. There is, we may believe,
a first phase of this process during which things are still
getting rapidly worse, during which the movement is
still in the direction of the paralysis or destruction of the
nerves concerned. It is with this phase that we may
correlate the initial terror or dread, which seems to occur
at the onset of any severe pain. There is a reaction, but
it appears as weak and helpless ; the mind seems to have
no resource available to stop the movement in the direction of yet more severe depression.[1] To this phase of

---

[1] " Fear is the anticipation of pain. For those forms of life capable
of fear this anticipation is not prevision, but a highly generalized fore-
feeling, itself unpleasant, that a yet more painful state impends. The
will to live, the élan vital, is more or less checked in its momentum or
narrowed in its range by some kind of intimation that it may be still
further held up." " Something bad has begun that is prelusive of
something worse." Stanley Hall, " A Synthetic-genetic Study of
Fear," *American Journal of Psychology*, Vol. 25 (1914), 149 and 152.

initial fear, often momentary, there will succeed normally a further stage of reaction in which a more definite attitude towards the unpleasant sensation is taken, and therewith the self more definitely separates itself from, and takes up a position towards, the sensation or its cause. This may take a weaker, less " sthenic " form, in which the dominant affective tone is still fear, a yielding or surrender to the unpleasant sensation, but there is active endeavour to terminate it by some form of avoiding movement. Or it may take the more sthenic form, in which the self asserts itself more strongly, and tending to treat the sensation as due to some hostile external cause, turns on the latter with the emotion of anger, which expresses itself in expelling or combating movements.[1] At the same time there occur certain further organic changes, affecting mainly the circulation, the heart's action, and the respiration, though so far as I know it has not been at present accurately determined how these differ in anger and in fear.[2] This description, however, is only likely to be fully true of cases of acute and abrupt unpleasure, such as those resulting from a severe bodily lesion. In cases of slight unpleasure, such as those which we have described as due to the over-stimulation of the sensory nerves, for example, a harsh or grating noise, a bitter taste, or a " crude " colour, we do not as a rule detect any trace, even the slightest, of fear emotion. Doubtless this is because the initial depression is very rapidly compensated by the reaction in these cases. But there is normally, I think, a slight emotion of anger, something which we describe by the term " irritation " or " annoyance ".

---

[1] I think the experiments in Wohlgemuth's *Pleasure—Unpleasure*, so far as they go, support this view. Anger, when due to the stimulus alone and not to some intellectual factor, tends as a rule to arise somewhat late in the course of the feeling process. When both fear and anger are mentioned, the former appears first and is succeeded by the latter, though sometimes a mixture of fear and anger is recorded. I can trace no report in which fear, due to stimulus only, is recorded as occurring after anger. Examples of the foregoing are W. 26, 50, 56, 113, 115, 139, 169, 170 ; Y. 180.

[2] Cf. on this point Cannon, *Bodily Changes in Pain, Hunger, Fear and Rage*, 280.

F

The actual happenings of ordinary life are, however, complicated in many ways by the pre-existing circumstances and state of the mind. What repeatedly happens is that a sensation, which taken by itself would be unpleasant, occurs when our attention is concentrated on some particular object or pursuit in which we are interested, or when for some other reason there already exists a dominant affective state or mood. In such circumstances the sensation may be noticed and recognized as unpleasant, but the normal emotional result of fear or anger does not occur. What happens here is doubtless this; the unpleasant sensation is present in consciousness together with the primary rejection involved in the unpleasure, but the dominant affective attitude is strong enough to prevent the rise of any other emotion involving an attitude of the self. This may happen in varying degrees according to circumstances. It is difficult to say whether fanatics or martyrs have always actually felt their tortures as unpleasant, or whether their enthusiasm may have been sometimes such that even the primary rejection due to the bodily reaction could be prevented from affecting consciousness. While the ordinary person has little guidance from his own experience in this matter, it would seem probable that if a sensation of pain is present at all, there is also felt the first stage of unpleasure together with primary rejection. In extreme cases of mental preoccupation no doubt the sensations of even severe bodily injury may be unnoticed at the time, as soldiers have been said not to notice wounds in the excitement of battle. In that event, however, not only the feeling but also the sensation is not present in consciousness.

What we have been describing hitherto is the earlier stage of pleasant or unpleasant experience. If the experience is further prolonged, there will occur varying changes of emotional and conative attitude. Initial fear or anger may be succeeded by a more passive attitude, that of " resignation ". Or the mere persistence of the unpleasant sensation may cause a return of fear. Further consequences may be entailed by the rise of associated ideas, caused by memories of the past, e.g. to the effect that bodily injury leads to further unpleasant consequences later, or by general ideas, which include principles of value. It is thus that from further reflection there arises for example that extreme condemnation and rejection of bodily pleasure which we find in ascetic philosophers; the expression of Antisthenes, " May I be mad rather than feel pleasure ", or that of Iamblichus : " The greatest of all evils is pleasure, because by it the soul is nailed or riveted to the body ".[1] But with this question of further valuation we may hope to deal again later.

Before we leave this part of our subject, it is as well to mention a quite recent theory of the feelings, which has attracted considerable attention and seems to have certain affinities to our own. W. M. Marston in his work *The Emotions of Normal People* has put forward the view that the mutual facilitation of any two motor impulses on a motor " psychon " constitutes conscious pleasantness ; antagonism between two or more motor impulses within any motor psychon constitutes conscious unpleasantness.[2] Apparently alliance or antagonism between any two simultaneous impulses can occur. But in the majority of cases, including those of the simpler sensory feelings (as usually so termed), the pleasure or unpleasure occurs because the motor impulses generated by a stimulus either reinforce or inhibit the constant " tonic " discharge by which the attitude of the organism and (presumably) its main functions are maintained. This theory plainly has affinities to that given above, but it also seems to me that as stated it must be judged inadequate. That impulse gives pleasure, it is stated, which facilitates or reinforces the constant motor discharge.

---

[1] Quoted by Lecky, *European Morals*, I, 326.
[2] Op. cit., 78. By the term " psychon " he means the synapses existing in the paths of motor discharge concerned.

But whence comes the reinforcement ? Marston is nowhere definite on this point. It is surely obvious that the tonic discharge is maintained by afferent or sensory impulses ; and that therefore its reinforcement can only come, in the case of the simple sensory feelings dealt with by us, from a reinforcement of the sensory process. That such a reinforcement of sensory processes is a fact in pleasure, it has been our object to show. In that case, however, it is in the sensory fact that is to be found the origin of the whole phenomenon ; and we shall be right to find in it the essence of the affective phenomenon. The motor facts must be secondary, the diffused results of the sensory process.

Let us pass to the case of unpleasure. Marston's view apparently is that the unpleasure arises because a very intense stimulus has very intense reflex effects, which conflict with the tonic motor discharge or with the pre-existing motor " set " of the organism, whatever it may have been.[1] This explanation, however, does not seem called for, even if we confine our attention for the moment to those cases of excessive stimulation which it is designed to meet. When we are interrupted in our existing occupation by an unpleasant sensation, there are two unpleasant-nesses which can be distinguished, that of the interruption, and that which seems to appertain to the sensation itself and would appertain to it more or less equally whenever it occurred. It is this latter which has to be explained ; for it cannot be due merely to the fact of interruption of pre-existing conscious occupation or tendency. If it is explained as due to motor conflict at all, the conflict must be one set up with the pre-existing tonic discharge by which the general attitude and pro-cesses of the organism are being maintained. On this point Marston gives some interesting observations, show-ing that indifference to a " painful " stimulus may be attained if the involuntary motor reactions which norm-ally occur in response to such a stimulus can be repressed ;

[1] See op. cit., 80 and 177.

and he suggests that this is the secret of many of the
marvellous achievements of Oriental adepts in enduring
bodily lacerations.[1] To a certain extent of course the
involuntary reaction to a painful stimulus acts remedially.
Writhings, groanings, etc., are experienced as a distraction
and a relief, and if while suffering we are prevented from
moving (e.g. in the dentist's chair) that fact does seem to
increase the intensity of the unpleasure. But we would
not wish to stress this point as an answer to Marston's
theory. We can agree that if *complete* absence of motor
reaction can be attained, the result may be abolition of
unpleasure ; for when we are suffering in the dentist's
chair and prevented from moving, there will probably
still be an intense contraction of the voluntary muscles
and tension of the whole bodily system in response to the
painful stimulus. The better explanation seems rather
to be on the same lines as that already given (see p. 66).
Normally an acutely unpleasant stimulus means a reaction and tension, which affects the whole organism and
carries therewith an attitude of rejection on the part of
the conscious self, and a striving to reinstate the normal
course of the bodily life. But if, as the result of some
motive derived from a higher mental stratum, it is possible to suppress the motor reaction, the process is cut
short at the point at which it passes into a fully conscious
unpleasure ; the attitude of the conscious self becoming
one of compliance and acceptance, and not one of rejection. We have already noted that this effect may vary
in accordance with the completeness and energy with which
the attitude of the conscious self can be maintained. In
extreme cases it is perhaps possible that, while some sensation yet remains, all trace of unpleasure may yet be
abolished ; but this is a point on which it is difficult to
obtain evidence from ordinary experience.

Doubtless neither the account given by us nor that
given by Marston can pretend to give a complete or de-
cisively acceptable account of the neural events. Both

[1] See op. cit., 60 and 179–81.

involve many hypothetical elements. No doubt the fact of obstruction of any impulse to motor discharge is a case of unpleasure, as we have already pointed out. But we can hardly do justice to the facts unless it be admitted that unpleasure is also the result of conflict or disturbance occurring in the sensory sphere of neural life. There is unpleasure due to deprivation of sensory stimulus, and of this, so far as I can see, no account is given in Marston's theory. There is also the acute unpleasure resulting from an impediment to repose or sleep. It would surely be impossible to show that when sleep is prevented there is a conflict between motor impulses. The most which it would be possible to show would be a conflict between a motor tendency set up by a stimulus on the one hand, and on the other a tendency towards relaxation or cessation of activity. This could hardly be brought within the scope of Marston's theory as stated by him.

The theory of the " motor self ", as it is termed by Marston, involves the concept of a stationary equilibrium, liable to be disturbed by phasic or temporary reactions. Any such disturbance is on this view likely to be initially unpleasant. We find in fact that Marston holds that the reaction to food does mean an alteration of the " natural reflex balance ".[1] As against this view we find it more natural to believe that the physical life consists rather in a moving equilibrium, which includes rhythms and alternations. It is surely an unnatural view of life which treats nutrition as disturbance.

[1] See op. cit., 217.

PART III

PLEASURE AND UNPLEASURE IN RELATION TO THE MAIN INSTINCTS

CHAPTER I

INSTINCTS OF NUTRITION AND BODILY MAINTENANCE

WE now pass to the consideration of what are ordinarily termed the separate instincts, and might be distinguished as such from those conations, hitherto described, which are directed to the maintenance and rejection of sensations. Our object in the first place is to see what is the connection of pleasure and unpleasure with the instincts, and in the second to decide whether, given that there are conations of different orders, occupying different places in the scale of development, there is a corresponding difference of quality or order between the feelings going with such conations. It is therefore necessary to describe the various instincts, and see whether it is right to designate any of them as " higher " in distinction from the bodily impulses, hitherto dealt with, which might be described as " lower ". We shall not in the first place endeavour to state any provisional principle of classification or distinction, but will proceed directly to examine the chief human instincts, taking those ordinarily so treated in present psychology.

To give a complete account it would be necessary to pass in review all the human instincts, and this, if fully carried out, would be a very lengthy matter. We shall hope to find that it is possible to isolate certain large groups and types of human instincts, in such a way that we shall be able to obtain an adequate view of the general nature of the instincts, and their relation to the feelings.

There are, of course, a number of instinctive actions, such as sucking on the part of the infant, which occur at once on the appropriate stimulus and are practically perfect from birth. Whatever may be the past history of development that has led to them, at present they are not accompanied by any noticeable feeling. An instinctive action of this nature is indeed not to be distinguished from the general class of automatic reflexes. The instincts which we propose to consider are those involving a more or less prolonged conative train, in which there is the possibility of success or non-success.

The most fundamental of all the animal instincts is usually considered to be that of food seeking. The vital activity of living substance consists essentially in the intake and absorption of nutritive matter and of oxygen, and in the giving outwards in exchange of the products of internal decomposition. Plants, inasmuch as they can draw nutriment from the inorganic, that is to say live in a constant nutritive medium, carry on this process continuously. Animals absorb oxygen continuously, but inasmuch as they are dependent on organic substances for food, their intake of such food must be intermittent. Originally, no doubt, animals were dependent on accident for coming in contact with nutritive material; when they came accidentally into contact with something capable of being absorbed and were also in need of food, they absorbed it, as is still the case with marine sedentary animals. From the first, so we have asserted, there has resided in the organism an effort to maintain its own proper vital processes. In the absence of food this effort expresses itself as a tension and restlessness, which has two constituents. In the first place there is the action of the special organ concerned, the stomach, which when empty contracts with increasing energy; a form of action which it is possible may be partly stimulated by a toxic product in the blood.[1] In the second place, there is the reaction by the organism generally against the general

---

[1] See above, p. 48.

incipient depression due to absence of nutrition. This tension and restlessness develop into the movements of food seeking. As the result of success and failure there further develop and become fixed as innate characteristics of different species, a vast number of auxiliary actions, such as responses to the distant effects of food substances, prey-catching contrivances, etc. All these can be nothing but differentiations of the original hunger restlessness, resulting from the struggle for survival in many varieties of circumstances. Many facts of animal life go to show that the connection between the craving of hunger and the distance effects of food substances (sight or smell) is not a mechanically predetermined matter, but learnt through experiences of success and failure, and that the governing factor is the satisfaction of the hunger craving. Lambs, says Hudson, will at first suck at any part of the mother's body and will often suck for a long time at a tuft of wool.[1] Chicks, as Lloyd Morgan showed, peck at first with perfect impartiality at any small object, grain, small stones, their own and companions' toes, etc., and only learn through experience to take the satisfying and reject the unsatisfactory.[2] A remarkable instance of the non-fixedness of food instincts is that given by the Kea parrot of New Zealand.[3] The food of this parrot up to the time of the introduction of sheep into the country had been grubs and roots. It suddenly and rapidly changed its habits and took to settling on the back of the sheep, and tearing it open so as to get at the kidneys and feed on them. This sudden change can only have been due to experience (originally no doubt accidentally acquired) of the greater satisfaction to the hunger craving given by this animal diet. It is probable that the process of acquisition of food habits is throughout a matter of trial and error, and that where reactions to the distance effects of food substances are innate, it is because success has led to

[1] Hudson, *Naturalist in La Plata*, 107.
[2] Ll. Morgan, *Habit and Instinct*, 40.
[3] See Finn, *Bird Behaviour*, 61, etc.

such reactions becoming established hereditarily in the species.

In man, living in organized society, the original impulse of hunger craving takes the form of the adoption of a trade or profession, with all the activities pertaining thereto. We have already remarked (in dealing with the sensory feelings) that moderate hunger is not unpleasant, but rather appears as adding a zest to the bodily life ; and that it only becomes unpleasant at a certain degree of acuteness. In proportion as nutrition has become intermittent, the alternation, within certain limits, between hunger and repletion has become part of the essential rhythm of life. And moreover, the food-seeking acts have become an essential part of the vital activity of the developed animal. For living animals in general to be supplied with food without any effort of their own means as a rule a great deterioration in the level of life ; and this would be applicable to the great majority of mankind. Among the races highest in intellectual development there are a number of persons who can, when no longer under the necessity of earning their own living, find occupation and enjoyment in some form of play, to use that word in its widest sense. But even for most of these such play takes the form of an imitation of earlier forms of food seeking, i.e. hunting and other kinds of sport. For those successfully earning their own living a great part of the pleasure felt is contributed by satisfaction of the impulse of self-assertion. The man who feels that he is filling a place in society as an equal among equals and contributing his share to the maintenance of the whole, derives therefrom a glow of pride or self-respect, which forms a permanent background in his experience ; while the failure and wastrel suffer proportionately from a sense of inferiority in relation to others. But these impulses belong to a higher level of mental life than that now in question. The maintenance of life in its full energy is in itself pleasant, and depression of vitality unpleasant. But the matter is not quite adequately described in these simple terms. It is of the essence of mind as we know it in ourselves to look forward into the future. He who is successfully maintaining life by his own activity, who feels himself adequate to the demands of self-preservation, looks forward to the future with hope and confidence. Conversely, when the level of vital activity is depressed, the looking forward tends to be anxiety and dread. We have already described this note of fear as existing at the onset of any acute bodily unpleasure. As a more permanent state of anxiety it tends to come into existence when the level of the bodily life is depressed by innutrition, that is to say when the trend of life seems downwards rather than upwards. The note of fear will be present to those who find themselves failing in the struggle for self-maintenance and therefore powerless to stay the downward progress of vitality; and it will be the most important factor in their unpleasure. This fear, which begins as an instinctive reaction of the conscious self to the organic sensations, becomes, when the self is fully aware of its meaning, that which we know as the conscious fear of death. But there could never arise such a conscious fear unless there were from the first an instinctive struggle against that lowering of vitality which points, as it were, to its complete destruction.

The food-seeking impulse is usually treated as a separate instinct. But it would appear that what is really here concerned is the maintenance of the bodily functions which are accompanied by the sensations of health and well-being. This maintenance is an essential part of life. We can rather consider as separate instincts those forms of tendencies to action which are auxiliary to the main-tenance of the bodily nutrition, such as direction towards a particular kind of visual or olfactory object which serves as food; and as auxiliary tendencies too may be considered a number of repulsions or aversions towards specific substances, which are accompanied by the emotion known as disgust. In the course of time many of these tendencies have become fixed in the different species as inherited instincts. We cannot be sure whether natural selection and accidental variation alone are sufficient to account for them, or whether any effects of a successful habit established in one generation are inherited by the next. This is a point which at present has to be left open. But whatever the cause, we know that somehow such separate instincts favourable to bodily maintenance have become hereditary. Among the auxiliary instincts too we must count a large number of separate tendencies in which the connection with bodily maintenance is more indirect, such as construction of traps for prey, construction of shelters, acquisition and storage of food articles, annual migrations in the direction of more favourable climatic conditions and more plentiful food supply. All such instincts must be held to be in their origin subsidiary to vital self-preservation, i.e. to the maintenance of the series of the bodily sensations. Higher mental operations such as recognition and analogical construction may be involved as part of the means towards this self-preservation, but are not essentially part of the end. Strictly speaking, therefore, food seeking in its primary form cannot be regarded as an instinct of a different or higher order than the impulse to discharge and maintain the normal vital functions, which carries with it the feelings of sensory pleasure and unpleasure, as already described. It would, however, appear that the instincts, originally subsidiary to this vital maintenance, may, when they acquire a certain independence, sometimes rightly be described as having ends of a higher order than a mere sensory fact. For instance, the instinct to construct a shelter will not only involve as its means varying effort and adaptation to difference of circumstances, but its end also is a fact of a somewhat higher order intellectually than a sensory fact, i.e. the creation of a complex perceptual situation, which will be a whole including relations.

There is, however, the germ of further development even in the simplest form of self-maintenance. The self-

maintaining effort of conscious life must at any stage
have been something more than the self-perpetuation of
a mere series of bodily sensations. There must always
have been a conscious unit as the centre of, and bond
between, these sensations, and not identical with them,
however closely it is bound up with them. In self-
maintenance it is this conscious unit whose existence is
prolonged into the future. Ultimately there comes into
existence at a later stage of intellectual development a
will to the preservation of a conscious self, fully conceived
as a continuing existence in relation with an external
world, and a conscious fear of death or annihilation.
This fully conscious self-preservative effort is the direct
outgrowth from the blind self-preservative impulse here
described. To this extent even the simplest form of
instinct, that directed to the maintenance of a simple
sensory fact, contains in germ the element of a relation
between the self and its objects.

When we pass to the further consideration of the
instincts, we shall find that, in a number of cases at least,
the instinctive impulse only attains its full development
gradually, by a process, as it were, of maturation. In this
process unpleasure does not necessarily play a part.
It is not the case that an unpleasant state of want gives
the initial impulse and that the agent learns gradually
what will satisfy that want and remove the unpleasure.
The picture that presents itself is rather that of an innate
capacity, which tends to unfold itself gradually, until the
full possibilities inherent in it are realized. This process
may be accompanied by pleasure throughout, though this
will vary in degree according as progress is more or less
equal, and will give way to unpleasure, if progress is at
any time held up by some impediment.

The first example we will take is that of the acquisition
of one of the chief means of locomotion. The actual
process of learning to walk by the child is a gradual one.
Initially at a certain stage of development there appears
a tendency, apparently reflex in character, to stiffen the

legs and press downwards as soon as the ground is felt, and also to move them in alternation.[1] But this does not lead to immediate perfect exercise of the function of walking with balance. Perfection is only attained as the result of effort and after some failures, the first attempts being made with the help of some outside support. James[2] has surmised that this is only due to the fact that the first attempts are made before the co-ordinating centres in the brain have quite ripened for their work ; and that if a child were kept from walking for a few weeks when the impulse first presents itself, he would be able to walk at the end of that time as well as if the ordinary process of " learning " had been allowed to occur. He supports this by an observation of Spalding's on young swallows, who were prevented from flying until fully fledged and then flew almost as well as the mature bird. I do not know whether James' surmise has ever been tested on a child. But the normal course of the actual events shows that something has been missed out, if this is to be taken as meant for a complete account of the matter. In the first place the fact of the existence of an implement is not identical with the fact of its use. And in the second place, in order to find out what is the inner essence of the use in this case, we are justified in inferring from our knowledge of the meaning of gestures and expressions in ourselves to what they mean in others. Thus we are able to believe that behind the efforts of the child to walk there is a physical factor, which may be described as follows : in the first place a vague restlessness which leads to the performance of the first sketch of locomotory movements, in accordance with the inherited structure, when the appropriate situation is present ; then a feeling of the incompleteness of such movements and effort to complete and perfect them, an effort at first only guided by a vague or semi-blind awareness of what is required,

[1] Preyer, *Mind of the Child*, I, 274 and 275. James, *Principles of Psychology*, II, 405.
[2] Loc. cit., 406 and 407.

but which gradually becomes more definite, as partial successes are attained through the random movements and are accompanied by feelings of growing satisfaction and pleasure. It would be wrong, I think, to ascribe the initial restlessness in any way to the spur of unpleasure. Stern, from the observation of his children, speaks of "living energy which craves for expenditure",[1] which finds its expression in all sorts of random movements as well as those of locomotion, and again of "unquenchable thirst for action".[2] Shinn, on the subject of the early movements of the child, writes as follows: "With the latter half of the first year came a period of peculiar pleasure in the movements of her body connected with the acquisition of the main race movements—rolling, creeping, standing, walking. In some cases the acquisition of these movements was sought very seriously, merely as a means to an end, and in others appeared accidental or almost automatic; but in still others it was attended with great joy in the exercise. On the whole, as her power over her body increased, her chief joy came to be in the free use of her muscles," i.e. the main instinctive movements, rolling, creeping, standing, walking.[3] And again on more general lines: "Besides the pure joy in existence that seemed to fill her, her pleasure in her own increasing freedom of muscular action and sense activity, her delight in motion and frolic, seemed to fill her days with an exuberant joyousness. Laughter, shouts of joy, overflowing ejaculations of happiness, deep and happy interest are constantly recorded in connection with special pleasures such as the use of her own bodily powers, exploring and investigating, etc. etc."[4] No doubt in all this there is mingled a purely sensory pleasure of general muscular exercise, derived, as we have already stated, partly from the activity of nerves which crave stimulation, and partly from the general increase of the activity of the

[1] Stern, *Psychology of Early Childhood*, 96.
[2] Op. cit., 309.
[3] Shinn, *Notes on Development of a Child*, I, 190.
[4] Op. cit., I, 239.

vital functions. But ordinary observation cannot fail to convince us also of the existence of a pleasure due to the successful completion of an instinctive effort, a pride of achievement, bound up with the realization of that perceptive content which we describe under the term " walking."

An instinct such as that just mentioned is perfected in a short time ; and afterwards its employment becomes a matter of constant habit and is not ordinarily accompanied by marked pleasure. We will now look at others whose development is more gradual.

CHAPTER II

THE REPRODUCTIVE INSTINCTS

WE will first consider the sexual instinct. Primarily the manifestations of sex in the living organism are a continuation of those of nutrition and growth. At a stage in the history of the organism growth ceases, and instead of growing further the individual separates off from itself cells which are capable themselves of growing into other living individuals. The foundation of the sexual impulses is thus to be found in a property of living substance as such. We cannot find in its origin any psychical factor, so far as we know. For all the higher animals the growth of the separated cells can only take place into new individuals through a sexual conjugation of such cells, i.e. through the union of the male spermatozoon with the female ovum. It is possible that the spermatozoon is attracted to the ovum of its own species by means of some special chemical substance diffused by the latter.[1] But we don't know whether such attraction could have any influence on the movements of the organisms while they are still acting as the carriers and protectors (to speak biologically) of the reproductive cells. We do know that for the individual there is the impulse to discharge these reproductive cells in such a way as to lead to their union with those of the other sex. This is secured by the fact that it is the perception of a certain object, namely the member of the other sex, which excites the impulse to discharge. It might be asserted that what we have here is only a reflex action excited by a certain sort of sensation ; it would be held that inasmuch as sexual discharge has occurred before in conjunction

[1] See Verworn, *General Physiology*, 433–6, and Tansley, *The New Psychology*, 219.

with the visual, tactual, or olfactory sensations due to the member of the other sex, these sensations acquire the power of causing sexual excitement in a preliminary and weaker form, just as it comes about that the salivary reflex is excited by the mere sight or smell of food. But I do not think this would be a correct description. In the first place that which excites the reaction is always an object, either a constellation of qualities or a simple quality; but in any case something perceived, i.e. treated as existing over against the agent and independent of it. In the second place that which is awakened by the object is a craving, not a mere reflex. The craving is shown in an incipient activation of the sexual organs pleasant in itself, but felt as incomplete and pointing on to the fuller activity. The physical conditions of this craving existed already in the form of the sexual maturation of the organism, and sometimes they may lead to some physical expression before the object is perceived. But normally the craving is only wakened to full activity by the perception. The craving is not only to discharge of the sexual function, but to its discharge in accompaniment with the perception of the given object, i.e. the member of the other sex. Only so can the impulse be fully satisfied. That this is so is a biological fact, which we must take as it is, and perhaps cannot further account for.

In the human race there is a certain potentiality of sexual desire with regard to any member of the opposite sex, but it is not as a rule aroused to activity except for some special reason. Whatever the reason may be, the attractiveness of some particular member of the other sex tends to be felt with especial force at one time and may dominate the total conscious life over considerable periods, becoming an enduring disposition or sentiment. There is a wider range of mental facts involved in this than mere sexual desire. There is in the first place a joy in the companionship of the beloved and unhappiness in absence. But this joy is not a merely passive and stationary thing.

It also passes over into a conation. The total conscious life of the beloved object appears to the agent as bound up with the exercise of his own pleasurable activity, and therefore as something precious and valuable ; it is at the same time realized with a peculiar vividness. The joy is in the companionship of a partner, existing in full vital energy. Not only, therefore, is there effort to preserve that conscious life intact, if there is any actual threat of injury to it ; but also, in virtue of the essentially prospective nature of the human mind, the agent assumes as it were an attitude of watch and ward against possible injury to the beloved, in advance of any actual threat. The conative energy of the lover goes out into a continuous attitude of protective tenderness. I suppose many persons, if asked what is the most perfect expression of tender emotion in literature, would be likely intuitively to give Heine's poem, " Du bist wie eine Blume." " You are like a flower, so beautiful and gentle and pure, I gaze upon you and sadness creeps into my heart. It is as though I ought to lay my hands upon you, praying that God may keep you so beautiful and pure and gentle." Analysing the poem we see that there is described in it exactly that course of feeling which we have mentioned, first an intense sympathetic realization of the beauty and value of the life of the beloved object, then premonitions of harm and the impulse to guard and keep intact. McDougall[1] has stated that there must be an innate connection bringing it about that in all save debased natures the object of the sexual impulse shall also become the object in some degree of tender emotion. It is perhaps doubtful whether the psychologist, as an observer, is justified in using the word " debased " with its implication of moral censure. But it is certainly the case that up to the present the family has been the normal mode of life for the human race ; and thus sexual desire on the part of the male without affection for, and with indifference to the future of, the partner and offspring does represent a decided

[1] *Introduction to Social Psychology*, 82.

deviation from the original norm. Such deviations can occur in the human race, because the pressure of the struggle for existence is so often mitigated. Amongst animals instincts are as a rule subject to little possibility of variation.

Sexual love is, however, of course more than just a selfless tenderness. There is included in it a demand for reciprocation. When it is known that love is returned there is assurance that the sexual desire will attain its full satisfaction. In addition to this, by the feeling that love is returned, self-feeling is heightened in several ways. It is highly gratifying to be preferred by one person above all the world and that by the one admired by oneself. The love of power is also gratified. " To have succeeded in gaining such attachment from and sway over another is a proof of power which cannot fail agreeably to excite the *amour-propre*." Sexual love is therefore, as Herbert Spencer has well pointed out,[1] a highly complex emotional state, and it owes to this fact a large part of its power. In it more than one of the innate tendencies of the human mind can find their realization and satisfaction.

All the feelings and impulses which we have described ripen as a rule gradually. There may be at first a gradual increase in the pleasantness of companionship with the beloved, which will pass unnoticed by the agent. The impulse towards sexual excitement exists, but only in a slight and incipient form, and therefore subconsciously. Very often what brings the gradually maturing tendency to consciousness is the shock of some disappointment or some impediment, for example, when an expected meeting does not take place, or when a possible rival appears. But this can hardly be necessary. It is possible that the maturing impulses may of themselves attain such power as to force themselves into consciousness without any such shock. It should not be necessary to point out that this total process may be pleasant throughout.

[1] H. Spencer, *Principles of Psychology*, I, 487–8, from which the foregoing is quoted.

It consists in the gradual maturation and working out of a conative impulse, which is only attended by unpleasure in so far as there is some obstruction to its progress. Obviously it would be absurd to think of the conative impulse as set in motion by the shock of the impediment or obstruction. It must have been in existence before.

. The conative train of which we speak reaches its first term in the actual fact of sexual intercourse, with its high degree of sensory pleasure. But it would not be right in my opinion to regard this as properly making a complete end in itself. It would be more correct to say that it marks the end of a stage in a total conative train, and that it leads on to a further process. Obviously this is so in the case of the female of the higher animal species. From the time of conception there begins as a rule some sort of preparation for the birth of the young ; it may be only the seeking of a hiding-place for parturition, or it may be the construction of a shelter, in which to rear the young. When the young are born, they are suckled or otherwise fed and protected. The length of time during which the young are dependent on the parent increases as the higher forms of animal life appear. Among many of the higher animals there is definite instruction by the parent in such activities as catching prey. The conative train is not worked out to its conclusion until the young are " placed out in the world " and able to support themselves. This process of development reaches its final term in the human race, in which the period of dependence is much longer than in any animal, and in which an enduring sentiment of affection tends to follow and endure throughout life. The question to be asked is whether the instinctive train terminates for the male with the act of sexual union. Tansley has said that, " The primary interest of the male in sex ends with the act of mating ".[1] It is true that there are great varieties in the animal world and it is difficult to say what is " normal " in this respect.

[1] Tansley, *The New Psychology*, 220.

The male in many species appears to have no interest in his partner after intercourse, nor *a fortiori* in the young. It has been asserted that young wolves are sometimes devoured by their fathers or older wolves, and have to be protected by the mother.[1] On the other hand it is a fact going very far back in the evolutionary history of the animal world that the male takes an instinctive interest in the female after intercourse and shares in the protection of the young. The males of some species of fishes and molluscs keep watch and guard on a particular female at the breeding season.[2] Among fishes indeed, when there is any parental care of the eggs at all, it is always (I believe) the task of the male ;[3] and we should probably be correct to connect this with the fact that among fishes the impregnation of the ovum takes place *after* it has been separated from the body of the female. When we come to higher animals similar facts are common. The male bird nearly always shares in the rearing of the young, and many species of birds pair for life. The larger carnivores frequently hunt in pairs and the male shares the task of bringing food for the young. Amongst herbivorous animals a very usual type of herd is that of a group of females, with their young, to which one male acts as leader and protector. We are not of course justified in believing that the male animal has any knowledge that the impregnated female is the bearer of seed which will develop into the future living individual. We can, however, believe that in the cases mentioned the male takes a continued interest in the female, not only as the source of sexual pleasure, but also with a certain prospectiveness of attitude. That is to say, the female is interesting as carrying the vague promise of some future development, and vague as this expectation is, yet it is not wholly indeterminate inasmuch as it is satisfied

---

[1] See Brehm, *Tierleben* (1915), *Säugetiere*, Vol. 3, 219–20. There seems, however, to be some dispute as to these facts.

[2] Schneider, *Der Tierische Wille*, 370.

[3] See Espinas, *Des Sociétés Animales*, 401, and Pycraft, *Courtship of Animals*, 181.

by the actual birth of the young, whom he later helps to feed and protect.[1] I do not know whether this view may be considered somewhat fanciful. Yet if paternal care for the young is instinctive in certain species, as seems to be the case, it seems probable that the gap between the time of impregnation and that of birth must be bridged in some such way. In the human race, owing to the long period of infancy, the assistance of the father is required for the support both of mother and offspring, and thus it must be considered one of the species in which the tendency to paternal care is innate. The basis of this instinct on the part of the father must be an interest, similar to that found in the animal world, taken in that living product separated from himself which contributes to the building up of a new individual. The interest is now made more definite because there is explicit knowledge of the causal sequence from the time of impregnation. But interest could not be created by the fact of abstract knowledge. There must be an instinctive disposition to such interest in the roots of human nature, and derived from the past history of the race.

Frequently no doubt, both by men and women sexual intercourse is regarded as an end in itself and not as an incident of a conative train which results in the birth of a new individual. I do not know whether among the higher animals, such as apes, such phenomena occur.[2] But generally speaking, in the animal kingdom sexual intercourse does result in birth, and it is restricted to certain definite periods of the year, which are usually such as to ensure the birth of the young taking place in the most favourable season, i.e. the spring. This restriction to a particular season disappears in man, and sexual impulses may arise freely at all seasons. There is thus, particularly in the human male, an overplus of sexual impulse, which results in intercourse which has no relation

---

[1] This mode of expression is based on Stout's treatment of instinct. See especially *Manual of Psychology*, 355.
[2] See Köhler, *The Mentality of Apes*, 313–15.

to birth. It would not be right to call this a "perversion". But it must be considered as a dissociation of one stage from the conative train to which it originally belonged, and its elevation into a separate end of value in itself. As we have seen, a similar phenomenon tends to occur in other instincts. That which was originally subsidiary may become an end in itself. As long as a surplus of vital energy really exists, its exercise in such a way can hardly be considered abnormal. We should only be justified in speaking of abnormality or perversion in case the end of the instinct were not being attained otherwise, that is to say, if consistent practice of intercourse with avoidance of procreation led to some form of "race suicide".

It is obvious that the carrying out of the instinctive train of actions leading to the rearing of the young is one that tends to maintain itself strongly, that it is accompanied by great pleasure, and that interruption or frustration means intense unpleasure and resentment, e.g. if there is any threat to the life of the offspring. There is, however, one point at which a remarkable exception seems to occur. Childbirth is a normal and necessary point in the series, and yet labour is accompanied by pangs of intense physical unpleasure. This seems at first sight to give a refutation of the view we put forward in dealing with the sensory feelings, namely, that the exercise of the normal bodily functions is accompanied by pleasure. The matter may, I think, be put in the following way. In the series of physical changes imposed by pregnancy, a point is reached at which the next stage cannot be accomplished without a severe strain on nerves and muscles otherwise not usually brought into use, i.e. those involved in the uterine contractions. The strain carries with it an over-stimulation of the nerves and therefore involves physical unpleasure. But the painful struggle is all the time tending to work itself out towards its natural termination in delivery ; and we can hardly help believing that always a certain mental pleasure underlies the physical suffering, a pleasure in the feeling of progress towards a normal end. From the biological point of view the unpleasure may moreover play a useful part ; for its diminution may act as a guide pointing towards the attainment of the end in delivery. We find other similar occurrences in the physical life, when the return to the normal involves unpleasant bodily strain, for example, the pain of returning circulation after frostbite, or perhaps the unpleasant strain of exercising long-disused muscles. In these cases what we find, I think, is that an unpleasure felt as imposed by the bodily constitution, and experienced as having a local centre and origin, is overlaid by a feeling of value or goodness, due to a fulfilled need, in which the conscious self is more deeply interested.

As in the case of the nutritive processes and bodily self-maintenance generally, so too in the case of the reproductive series a large number of subsidiary activities grow up in the course of racial history. Such are acquisition and storage of food supplies, construction of shelters for the young, etc. It is not necessary to go into these in detail. There is always a possibility that these instincts will acquire a certain independence, and yield some satisfaction in themselves apart from the reproductive tendencies to which they were originally subsidiary.

CHAPTER III

CURIOSITY, OR THE IMPULSE TO KNOWLEDGE

WE now propose to consider an impulse often not thought to be instinctive in the same way as those already dealt with, I mean that which makes for a more complete knowledge of the external world. It has indeed been usually recognized that there is such a thing as an instinct of curiosity. But the connection of this with the more developed forms of the human desire for knowledge has not always been admitted. In discussing this question we can hardly hope to give a complete account of the development of the cognitive processes. We shall, I hope, find it sufficient for our purposes to confine ourselves in the main to that aspect of them which concerns the classification and naming of objects. Even so a treatment at some length will be demanded.

The mental life, there can be no doubt, begins with awareness of difference or of change. There is no cognition except of change between two presented contents. "Semper idem sentire et nil sentire ad idem recidunt." Every difference or change does in its degree cause a jar or shock to the mind, which varies in degree with the extent of the transition involved. This shock of transition is, in my opinion, experienced as an affection of the self, as we can see when we contrast it with the opposite self-state, that involved in recognition. Suppose that a sensation occurs of a certain shade of colour or of a light, and then after a short interval of darkness the same colour recurs, there is a feeling which we can only describe as being " at home with " the sensation, of being adapted to it. Or similarly if after seeing a colour in one part of the visual field, one comes across it again after traversing a short neutral space. It is no doubt easy to imagine a physical substratum for this feeling in the fact that, the nervous elements having been once excited in a certain way, a similar excitation soon after finds them adapted and the current runs more easily. But this is more or less guesswork ; whereas the feeling of familiarity is something which can be observed. According to the observations carried out under experimental conditions by Katzaroff, recognition is primarily an affective and not an intellectual process, and depends on the fact that the given sensation, having occurred in consciousness before, has become associated with the feeling of the ego, has been, so to speak, enveloped by it.[1]

The feeling of familiarity or recognition can occur even with the simplest sort of sensation, such as a shade of colour, from which all influence of shape or pattern is as far as possible excluded.[2] But when we pass to cases of form and pattern, the facts stand out clearer. The apprehension of every form, however simple, means that a whole has to be grasped with the relations of its constituent parts. There must be an outline involving proportions of sides and of the total magnitude, diameter, etc., and the apprehension of this is a process, however short. Among forms and patterns, as soon as we pass beyond the very simplest, we find that there are some easier to attend to as wholes than others are. An irregular shape, one in which the sides and angles vary without any fixed plan, is much more difficult to apprehend than a regular or equiangular figure in which the same angles and proportions are repeated.[3] There must be a certain

---

[1] Katzaroff, *Archives de Psychologie*, Vol. XI (1911), summary of conclusions, 75–8. It is true that both Katzaroff and Claparède, in the additional note appended, distinguish recognition, as the recurrence of something already belonging to the ego, from the feeling of facilitation in the motor or intellectual reaction (p. 83). But it seems to me that the feeling of facilitation must be the most important element in the self-state involved in familiarity, and it probably comes before any reference to the past going with a completed recognition.

[2] See Lehmann's experiments on recognition of simple colours, *Philosophische Studien*, Vol. 5, 115–32.

[3] See Groos, *Spiele der Menschen*, 75. As the result of tests the preference by a child of five for the regular figure with straight lines was clearly shown.

minimum of internal differentiation in order that a pattern
may exist at all. But this being given, the pattern easiest
to grasp as a whole is that in which there is repetition in
a regular order. It is easier to sum up in thought such
a figure than an irregular one ; and consequently there is
in face of it a feeling of ease and power, as contrasted with
a certain bewilderment and impotence in face of the
irregular. The effort of the mind is from the first towards
an ease of attention in relation to objects, and it is aware
of its effort as baffled by that which it cannot grasp.

There is the same result of ease and power when forms,
which have once been apprehended, recur, even though
they may be intrinsically less regular. We may contrast
it with a certain bewilderment and distress which is shown
in quite early childhood before new forms. " Here it is
the nose preparing tracts for the eye, the eye preparing
them for the mouth, the mouth preparing them for the
nose again ", says James (in physiological language)
speaking of the recognition of faces.[1] Faces are in fact
almost the earliest sort of object which the young child
shows signs of recognizing. " Long before the 30th week
healthy children distinguish human faces definitely from
one another, first the faces of the mother and nurse, then
the face of the father, seen less often ; and all three of
these from every strange face."[2] At about the same time,
according to Preyer, there are signs of recognition of the
customary surroundings. If the infant in the period from
three to six months is brought into a room he has not
before seen, his expression changes, he is astonished. The
new sensations of light, the different apportionment of
light and dark, arouse his attention, and when he comes
back to his former surroundings, he is not astonished.[3]
Stern gives instances occurring at a somewhat later age,
about $1\frac{1}{2}$ years, in which children, brought back to their
old rooms after a short absence, showed unrestrained
delight in recognizing them.[4] In the earliest form of

---

[1] James, *Principles of Psychology*, I, 675.
[2] Preyer, *Mind of the Child*, Part II, 6.   [3] Preyer, loc. cit.
[4] Stern, *Psychology of Early Childhood*, 217.

such recognitions we can no doubt hardly imagine that there is any definite expectation that, given any part of the whole, the rest will follow in the same order as before. All that we need suppose is that, given the same sequence, the initial items with their interrelations have in some sort prepared the mind for those that will follow, which thus come as familiar, and that there thus results a feeling of ease in perception accompanied by pleasure, as contrasted with the bewilderment caused by new forms. Animals no doubt possess something of a feeling of familiarity and ease in their accustomed surroundings. If a new piece of furniture is introduced into a room, it will be found that the cat will as a rule go up to it and give it a brief exploration, thereafter apparently dismissing it to form part of the customary and unattended-to background of its life. And McDougall has described how a horse will alternately approach and flee from a strange object such as a coat on the ground.[1] We must, however, be content to leave it doubtful whether in this there is any seeking of the purely intellectual satisfaction of ease of attention, or whether in these cases the animal is motived by nothing but the need for security, a security which is felt in the customary surroundings and disturbed by the novel. In the case of the child, however, though there may be in the beginning a certain feeling of security in the accustomed, the whole course of development shows that there is also at work an impulse towards a purely cognitive or intellectual satisfaction.

Forms do not of course occur in isolation. They occur only against a background from which they have to be separated out, if they are to be attended to as wholes. In the earliest history of the child there are certain movements of a reflex character which prepare the way for selective attention to single objects, for example the tendency, probably reflex, to transfer the point of brightest light from marginal to foveal vision, and a similar tendency with regard to a moving object. But, as Stern has pointed

[1] *Introduction to Social Psychology*, 58.

out,[1] this by itself could not account for the persistence with which single objects or sounds are attended to, when once noticed, and for the signs of interest combined with the concentrated attention. It is impossible not to believe there is in the mind an innate need to isolate objects for attention, a need which doubtless as a rule does not act effectively unless some cue is first given by the actual arrangement of the patterns with which sensation provides us, and by such factors as their movement as a whole. Without some such selective attention our impression of the outside world would be nothing but a confusing blur. We know in our own experience that if we are placed before such an object as a wall-paper with an intricate pattern, and have nothing else to do (as when lying ill), we seem almost inevitably led to try and pick out the scheme by isolating certain forms from the confusing whole. A more striking example still is that given by the rhythmizing tendency in respect of sounds. When any series of sounds follows at regular intervals, for example the ticking of a clock, we find that as we listen to it we are breaking it up into separate rhythmic units, something like the feet of a line of poetry. In this there is involved both the separation from the uniform whole of units made up of two or three beats, with an interval between each unit, and also the ascription of an internal differentiation to these units. The internal differentiation of each unit, in addition to the mere separation of units from the mass of the whole, has the result of facilitating attention. Obviously it is easier to effect a separation between a series of trochaic feet ($-\smile$) than between feet each of which is composed of equal and unvarying parts, such as the spondee ($--$). This deep-seated need for clearly defined wholes to which to attend is, we cannot avoid believing, operative throughout mental life ; and is at least one factor which leads to the apprehension of the world as made up of separate things. It is not possible to hold that what is effective here is nothing but the limita-

---

[1] *Psychology of Early Childhood*, 104–6.

tion of the power of attention, i.e. that we attend to limited wholes for the sole reason that the amount we can grasp in one act of attention is limited. If this were so, why should the mind, of its own accord, go out to discover separate unities, where none are given by objective fact ?

The background from which the form, which is at the moment the object of attention, is separated out does of course continue to exist for the mind. " Whatever may be the special items with which the mind is occupied at any moment they are never apprehended as absolutely self-complete and self-contained. They are always apprehended as partial constituents of a whole which includes and transcends them and as connected with other unspecified constituents of the whole ".[1] The mind has a need to establish order and definiteness for this whole with its interrelated parts, as for the smaller wholes of which it is composed. Opposite a field of perception any part of which is indefinite or blurred, the mind does not function freely. There is an impulse towards fuller exploration of that which is indistinct, in order as far as possible to get rid of the vagueness and establish the whole as one in which the relations and outlines are able to be clearly apprehended. This is obviously the case in the spatial sphere.

More interesting from our point of view are the relations formed between ideas and dependent on memory, and it is these which we will now consider from the point of view of development. Forms as apprehended and retained in memory by the growing mind are certainly very vague and schematic in character. Such as they are, when known by the child sufficiently to be recognized, they begin to be associated with one another, and when two have occurred together more than once, the occurrence of one will lead to the expectation of the other. Such expectations begin very early in life. We may quote examples from Stern.[2] A child at $4\frac{1}{2}$ months old begins

[1] Stout in *Mind*, N.S. 77, Jan. 1911, 5.
[2] *Psychology of Early Childhood*, 110–11.

to part her lips and hold her head straight in anticipation of the spoon containing broth, which she sees coming to her lips, and about the same age she protests by struggling against the washing of her face with cold water, when she sees the sponge brought near, and so on. On the subject of association many views have been held, and we can only give here that view which we propose to adopt, ignoring others.[1] When a mental content A recalls another content B because they have occurred together in the past, what is effective in the recall is A regarded as a universal, i.e. A regarded as identical in content in the two cases. As events in time both A and B are particular and once past can never recur. But what is effective is the fact that A has an identical content at each time and that this is able to reinstate B, with which it was contiguous before, the B that recurs being also identical in content with the previous B. There occur cases of emergence of ideas into consciousness, not known at the time to be due to an association, but which, it may be afterwards discovered, must have been called up by their connection with some idea or sensation already present in the background of consciousness.[2] It has, moreover, been found that under special conditions, e.g. when hypnotized or by automatic writing, persons can, when asked, give descriptions of objects previously present to them but not attended to (e.g. in marginal vision), without there being any knowledge for the main conscious stream that they have seen the objects before.[3] It is not possible to say that there is a universal present or effective in these cases, inasmuch as there is no recognition, however faint or vague, of the identity of the past and present contents. The only account of the causal sequence that could be given would be one based on physiological

[1] What follows is in the main derived from Bradley's *Principles of Logic*, I, 34–7 and 299–345.
[2] Interesting examples of this in Freud, *Psychopathology of Everyday Life*, 315–18, Samuel Butler's *Note Books*, 65, Jerusalem in *Philosophische Studien*, Vol. 10 (1894).
[3] See Morton Prince, *The Unconscious*, 49–59, for examples.

connection between nerve centres. Where however there is some consciousness of recognition, the universality may be present for consciousness with different degrees of explicitness. Animals are capable of expectations based sometimes on similarity of form of a somewhat abstract character. This can be seen in the use and adaptation of tools by monkeys recorded by observers such as Hobhouse, Köhler, and others. Or to take an instance from more natural conditions, we find the following recorded by Darwin ; that dogs when crossing a desert country rushed down into the dry hollows of the ground looking for water ; " the animals behaved as if they knew that a dip in the ground offered them the best chance of finding water ".[1] The description " dip in the ground " here covers a number of instances only resembling one another in a very abstract manner. We do not suppose that in these cases there is any clear awareness of the identity of the different instances in respect of the essential form. Nevertheless recognition and the use of the element identical in the different instances must be considered to have been present. Whenever, so we hold, there is awareness of a recall as due to a connection established in the past, then there is awareness of identity, and not only is a universal implied, but also there is actually present a general idea of a rudimentary kind. The history which we shall try to trace is that of how the implicit general idea becomes clearly known as the universal which is a class including different instances.

It is beyond the scope of this work to go into the question of how far animals may possess articulate ideas of the past. Leaving this doubtful, it is our concern to try and trace the development of the universal idea or concept in the human mind.[2] We gave above some instances of expectations due to memory formed in very early childhood. In the instances given the expectations

---

[1] Darwin, *Descent of Man*, 116.
[2] As will appear, the facts of the course of development are chiefly based on Stern's *Psychology of Early Childhood*.

H

were all formed under the influence of some other instinctive need, such as hunger or thirst. The interest of the human development from our point of view is that expectations soon begin to occur, not because of a pre-existing need for satisfaction of some organic want, but for what we can only call purely theoretical reasons. We cannot go here into all the various ways in which this is shown. One of the most important is of course the expectation of confirming one sense by another, sight by touch, or hearing by sight, which plays its part in leading to the knowledge that the source of various sensations may lie in one external "thing". The point which we wish to consider specially is that of the attachment of names to things. One of the most important associations formed in childhood is that between the perception of an object (a special form) and a certain sound, which the child first receives as an auditory sensation and then finds it can itself produce. When the same or a similar object is perceived again, the sound previously heard in connection with it is suggested and used again. What is effective in bringing this about is for the most part its general scheme or shape ; and this, as we have said, implies that an element, identical in the two instances, is made use of as a universal. Children apply, and take delight in applying, the same name to objects which resemble each other, though at first the resemblance is often only vague and schematic. Thus "A little boy aged 2 years and 5 months on looking at the hammers of a piano which his mother was playing called out ' There's owlegie ' (diminutive of owl). His eye had instantly caught the similarity between the round felt disc of the hammer divided by a piece of wool, and the owl's face divided by its beak ".[1] " Romanes states that a child that was beginning to talk, saw and heard a duck on the water and said ' quack '. Thereafter the child called on the one hand all birds and insects, and on the other all liquids, ' quack '. Finally it called all coins also ' quack ', after having seen an eagle on a French

[1] Sully, *Studies of Childhood*, 29.

sou."[1] Sometimes no doubt the object of this extension
of the use of names is to get other instinctive needs
satisfied, as, for instance, in the case of a child who, as
related by Preyer, adopted the word "appn", from
apple, for all forms of food, thus signifying the fact of
hunger.[2] But numberless other instances show how the
children continue to extend use of words, for no apparent
reason other than the pleasure of doing it. We cannot
doubt what is the inner meaning of this. A certain
form has been apprehended, even if it be only vaguely.
On perceiving another form there is satisfaction in feeling
it is something that the subject is " at home with ", not
bewildered and baffled by. The application of the same
name, at first perhaps only a sign that the object *has been*
recognized, later becomes a help towards the feeling of
familiarity, ease, power. As soon as, in consequence of
an identity however partial, the same name is applied,
the subject can feel that the object is " ticked off ", is
something with which it knows how to deal. We may take
as an example a quotation which Stout makes from Stir-
ling ; though it belongs to a later stage of mental development than that of the child, it clearly illustrates the same
mental process. When Crusoe and Friday both saw the
ship, " what it was, was evident at a glance to Crusoe. . . .
In short, what to Crusoe was *an* object, was to Friday
only a dark and amorphous blur, a perplexing, confusing,
frightening mass of details which would not collapse
and become single and simple to him ".[3] To one situated
as Crusoe was, undoubtedly at the first suggestion of what
the object might be, or at the first glimpse of a part of it,
such as a mast and sail, the word " ship " would flash
before his mind ; and this would give the clue for the
rest of the details of the object and its general form, over
which the mind would then pass easily, having acquired
with the help of the word a pre-notion of the whole, while

---

[1] Preyer, *Mind of the Child*, II, 91. Many other instances could be
given ; e.g. Sully, *Studies of Childhood*, 163, 421-2, 424.
[2] Preyer, op. cit., II, 97.
[3] Stout, *Analytic Psychology*, II, 110-11.

incidentally it would also give a clue to the further associations of the object and its place in the scheme of things. Though no doubt this is a more complex case than the recognitions of children, it does give us a notion of the sort of satisfaction achieved by the child in applying the same name to objects of similar form. The great pleasure which this sort of recognition, together with the application of a known name, gives to children aged two and over, is well exemplified also in looking at pictures. The mere fact that pictures are not only coloured patterns but are meant to represent real objects, has of course first to be learnt. When this has been achieved, there is endless joy in picking out the representations and giving names to the objects recognised. Obviously this is purely theoretical in character. " The great joy which the child takes at the beginning of the second year in pictures is indeed a proof how, in addition to sensori-motor activity, the first beginnings of a higher form of activity, the contemplative, are showing signs of life ; the immediate transmutation of sight perception into movement is checked, and what has been seen can be subjected to mental consideration."[1] Of the inner nature of this pleasure other observers have no doubt ; it is essentially a pleasure of heightened power. "The little ones already love to look at pictures. They often enjoy the pictured thing more than the real one. The little observer calls out ' House ' joyfully, when he recognises one in a sketch, while he scarcely deigns to glance at a real one. Does this rest on the joy of solving the pictured riddle, while the real object gives him nothing more to guess ? . . . In these words it appears plainly that in the pleasure of recognition it is really a matter of joy in power, in the overcoming of a difficulty."[2] To which we may add this from Shinn. " The interest shown by the little ones in these recognitions is endless. At first it seems to be simply

---

[1] Stern, op. cit., 182.
[2] Groos, *Spiele der Menschen*, 156 (partly quoted from Sigismund), translated.

a joy in perceiving the resemblance, something akin to their joy in fitting concepts with names. There is a deep and primitive delight to the child, from the earliest synthesis of the senses, in bringing a whole range of perceptions into parallelism with another range."[1] We may observe that in most cases, particularly where recognition of " form " is involved, the process described must include an analysis, or abstraction, of some feature of a total perception, before it can be recognized and named in other surroundings. The little boy who, as described by Sully,[2] applied the name " Gee gee " to the drawing of an ostrich and to the model of a stork, because the length of the neck in each case bore some resemblance to that of the horse, must have analysed out from the figure of the horse an aspect of its shape which happened to impress him, arbitrary and vague as the selection may have been. As we have already pointed out, abstraction need not occur in the simplest cases of recognition ; but it is a general feature of all form recognitions, where the objects are at all complex. Analysis or abstraction of a feature of a given whole is then part of the same process which includes the extension of form-recognition to wider classes of objects, and with it there will go a constantly increasing accuracy of the attention to details of the shape abstracted. This process will be accompanied by an increased feeling of mental agency, and of power and certainty in dealing with the perception of the external world, as the recognitions made are constantly confirmed.

An important step in development occurs at or shortly after the age of two. At first names are only applied as suggested by the objects, though there is pleasure in applying them. Before an object as yet unnamed the child now begins to feel there is something wanting. There comes the felt need for a name, which shall, as it were, sum the object up and enable it to be easily placed and related to other known objects. The child, we may say, goes out to obtain that sense of ease and power which

---

[1] Shinn, op. cit., II, 183.　　　　[2] Op. cit., 424.

hitherto has only come to it incidentally. In other words, the child realizes, practically though not explicitly, that every object should have a name. The name of everything is incessantly asked. Stern describes "the unwearied search for names" which occurs at this period.[1] Of especial interest from our point of view is the story of this step in development as made by Helen Keller and Laura Bridgman, the two blind and deaf, and therefore dumb, children.[2] Helen Keller had at the age of about $1\frac{1}{2}$ years completely lost the senses of sight and hearing owing to illness. Subsequently, and before her eighth year, she had automatically and mechanically learnt to connect certain actual signs with certain objects, but had got no further. This is her own account, from memory, of how at the age of eight she suddenly realized that every object should have a name. "As the cool stream gushed over one hand she (the teacher) spelled into the other the word 'water', first slowly then rapidly. I stood still, my whole attention fixed on the motion of her fingers. Suddenly I felt a misty consciousness as of something forgotten—a thrill of returning thought, and somehow the mystery of language was revealed to me. I knew then that 'water' meant the wonderful cool something that was flowing over my hand. That living word awakened my soul, gave it light, hope, joy, set it free. . . . I left the house eager to learn. Everything had a name and each name gave birth to a new thought. As we returned to the house, every object which I touched seemed to quiver with life. That was because I saw everything with the strange new sight that had come to me."[3] What distinguishes this from the ordinary course of development is that owing to her physical disability the child was unable to communicate easily with others,

---

[1] Op. cit., 163.

[2] This history in the case of Helen Keller is used by Stern to illustrate the same point (op. cit., 163). He quotes Miss Sullivan, the teacher. I have ventured to quote Helen Keller's own description, given from memory, as at least purporting to give an account of the experience from the inside.

[3] Helen Keller, *Story of My Life*, 23–4.

continually asking questions and getting replies, as an ordinary child would, and the normal development was thus held up. When the difficulty was removed, the normal development of ideas was, as it were, telescoped into a brief period and was completed with great rapidity. The pleasure ordinarily felt in the gradual expansion of power was concentrated into this brief period and intensified. Moreover, owing to its late occurrence, the child was able to remember and record her feelings. What is undoubtedly a similar moment of achieved insight is recorded by the teacher of Laura Bridgman, whose history is like that of Helen Keller. " At times," her teacher writes of this period, " she was too radiant with delight to be able to conceal her emotions."[1]

The discovery, thus described above, does not however necessarily mean that universals are now fully apprehended as classes which include a number of particular instances. As the same name is applied often to similar objects, there comes to be an increasing awareness of the past instances as past and distinct from the present instance ; and this is helped by the growing power of language in general to formulate memories of the past. There is a stage in which the child knows that a " horse " is met with not once only, but in many instances, which he marks by the application of the same name ; but he only makes statements about each particular horse. He forms objects into groups by counting " one more ", " one more ", and so on, or numbers them ; but he does not grasp the idea of the last-named number as the general summarized term for all the objects enumerated. Stern calls this the stage of " plural ideation ".[2] A good instance

<hr>

[1] See pp. 51–3, *Life of Laura Bridgman*, Howe and Hall. It is true that Dr. Howe considers the joy shown as entirely due to the child feeling she had now the link of language by which to communicate with others. No doubt this factor may have entered into the child's ideas. We should not forget that in our account we are isolating one feature of a complex process of mental development. I think the facts cited by us show the feeling of expanding power of intellect must also be a factor.

[2] Stern, op. cit., 378–81, from which the above is taken.

given by Stern is that of a child aged 3½, who asked
if a certain bird lays eggs, and was answered, " Yes, all
birds lay eggs ". But inasmuch as this generalized statement had no meaning for her, she went on asking " Does
this one lay eggs too ? " and failed to understand the
answer given to each question, " Yes, all birds lay eggs ".[1]

From this stage, which, as we have already stated,
implies the presence of a general idea or concept, though
not in a fully developed form, it is not difficult to see how
the transition occurs to the explicit concept. If a number
of perceived objects can be counted separately, and then
included under one designation, such as five bricks or five
persons, there is present something which serves as a
model for the idea of a general class which includes
a number of particular instances. It is towards the end
of the fourth year, according to Stern, that questions are
asked or other remarks made which include the use of the
collective " all ". Here is an instance given by Stern.
A boy aged 4 years 10 months was asked how many
fingers he had. On his answering " ten ", he was asked
how many his nurse and mother had, and answered
" ten " in each case. " Well then ? " asked his mother.
And in slow deliberation came the answer. " Then
. . . everybody has ten fingers ". But earlier than this,
during the 4th year, questions had been asked including
the use of " all ", such as " Do all horses have a white
spot ? " "Are there glasses like that in all cupboards ? "[2]

There is a theory which has attempted to describe the
formation of concepts by what James has termed the
" law of dissociation by varying concomitants ". " What
is associated now with one thing now with another tends
to become dissociated from either and to grow into an
object of abstract contemplation by the mind."[3] To
symbolize this process the following diagram (on the
opposite page) has been constructed " from which C
' rolls out ', an abstract idea in quasi-isolation ready

---

[1] Stern, op. cit., 403-4.   [2] Stern, op. cit., 404.
[3] James, *Principles of Psychology*, I, 506.

for recombination in all possible ways ".[1] This theory has been destructively criticized;[2] and certainly it is impossible that a general or universal idea could be generated in this way. It would be a process similar to that of composite photography, in which a number of images are superimposed, with the result that only the features common to all the images are preserved and those peculiar to each are eliminated. But in fact the result in such a case would only be another particular image with some of its details rather blurred, and not the idea of a class. As Lotze pointed out long ago, by a process such as that imagined the individual ideas in balancing

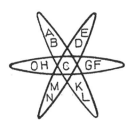

one another would disappear and be lost, whereas in truth they continue to exist ; the universal would not be felt as universal, as true of them amongst others, if they had vanished and simply left it behind as their production.[3] Moreover the fact that a given quality or shape occurs oftener than others and in conjunction with less frequent and varying concomitants would never by itself result in the idea of a universal, if the materials are regarded as each merely particular. If so, the formation of a general idea would be something accidental, depending on the number of times a given quality happened to recur. The law of varying concomitants would only be another way of saying that ideas of classes are formed because

[1] Carveth Read, "Relations in Thought," *British Journal of Psychology*, IV (1911), 350. But how far Carveth Read considers this as the source of general concepts I am not sure. He is speaking more immediately of abstraction.

[2] See McDougall, *Outline of Psychology*, 381.

[3] Lotze, *Metaphysic*, 477, § 272.

there are in fact resemblances in external nature. On the other hand this law might be stated in the following form : Suppose that in every case of recognition there is in fact, as stated above, at work an implicit idea of identity, or of a universal ; then every time that a similar recognition is repeated, it might be alleged that the idea of the constantly recurring quality is strengthened, and owing to this predominance it becomes a separate object for attention, until it gives rise to the explicit idea of an identical quality which recurs, the emergence of this idea being of course helped by the repetition of the same name through association. This account, which is one of how an implicit idea of identity becomes explicit, would be not dissimilar to that which we have given in the preceding. But what seems to be wanting in it is any sufficient reason why repeatedly attention should be paid to the respects in which concrete objects are like each other rather than to those in which they differ from one another. As James himself points out, it often seems to be rather the differences from the familiar that attract attention.[1] Often there is no attempt to trace out resemblances in the external world, but in as far as any feeling is present at all, there is a delight in the mere variety of the world, in its concrete richness. But though this is a fact in mental life, it is certain that it is by reason of other factors that intellectual advance is achieved. In our view the explicit drawing out of the idea of a class or universal proceeds in two ways. Firstly as the result of practical needs. Whenever, as we have said, a generalized expectation is formed as the result of previous experience, and this is acted on, in order to supply some bodily need, the idea of a universal is implied. It will be of advantage to the agent to be able to formulate rules of this sort explicitly in verbal form. If, to take the example already quoted, a man is able to say, " All depressions in the ground, especially those with other qualities such as presence of vegetation, are likely to contain water ",

[1] Op. cit., I, 507.

he will be able to store up a far greater number of such useful rules than the animal can ; moreover he will be able to include in them a more accurate statement of the exact conditions under which water is found, and he will also have the advantage of being able to obtain such general information from his fellows and to communicate his knowledge to them. In such a case as this the motive under which the mental advance takes place is the satisfaction of a bodily need or the will for self-preservation. A number of general rules, including concepts, have thus come to be formulated by the human mind, and we may assume that the main factor in the racial development of intellectual power has been the selection of those races who have been most capable of planning ahead and formulating their plans in detail for practical needs. But the history of human development seems to show that the formation of concepts is also due to another form of mental activity, which may however have emerged later in racial history. We have endeavoured to describe above the effort by the child to master its surroundings in thought, to pass from obscurity and bewilderment to clearness, certainty and power, and it is under the influence of this impulse that it is led to emphasize or pay attention to those aspects in which objects resemble one another. There is of course a common stock of general ideas, acquired in nearly equal measure by all the minds in a given society. This is embodied in the current language of the time and handed down by teaching to the younger generations. Without such teaching the child would not attain to it. A child brought up by animals (as in the alleged cases of wolf-children in India) would have made no steps towards it ; and the experience of a European child brought up by savages might be organized very differently from what it is. The point of our description has been to show that, in the process of acquiring this stock, the spontaneous effort by the child towards mastery of its surroundings in thought does co-operate. In the past history of the race too this impulse, together with practical needs, must have contributed to build up the stock of general ideas embodied in our language ; though it is not possible here to go into the racial history, or the question of origin, that must lie behind.

In order to define the nature of this impulse further another point must be emphasized. It might be supposed that the mind in seeking for generalizations is acting under a principle of " economy ", as it has been called. On this view, as the span of our attention is limited, and external objects are infinitely diverse, it affords a relief to comprehend them under unities, as few as possible. The impulse to find unity would then be only a sign of our mental limitation, and though the mind would still be conceived as active, its endeavour would only be to avoid fatigue and overstrain.[1] But this account would not do justice to the facts. If it were true, intellectual satisfaction would consist in attending to one undifferentiated object at a time, and the nearer approach to blankness the greater the satisfaction. The mind in truth seeks exercise and not only economy. Sometimes the external world is too uniform for it, and we have the unpleasant feeling of monotony. The mind does not rest content either with an undifferentiated unity or with a disconnected manifold. The grasp of attention is of course limited. But within those limits the mind aims at comprehending the greatest possible number of apparent diversities under as few general laws as possible. The greater the number of objects or events which it can thus survey under one aspect, the greater its feeling of power and the higher its satisfaction. This we shall see exempli-

---

[1] This view may be combined with a pragmatic theory of the nature of intelligence. Thus James writes as follows : " My thinking is first and last and always for the sake of my doing, and I can only do one thing at a time. A God, who is supposed to drive the whole universe abreast, may also be supposed, without detriment to his activity, to see all parts of it at once and without emphasis. But were our human attention so to disperse itself, we should simply stare vacantly at things at large and forfeit our opportunity of doing any particular act " (*Principles of Psychology*, II, 333). But whether this is consistent with his view of classification logic and mathematics as resulting from the " mere play of the mind in comparing its conceptions " (see p. 659) may perhaps be doubtful.

fied in looking at the later developments of the intellectual impulse.

We have endeavoured already to trace the development leading to the first formation of general ideas. It is about from this time that there begins in the life of the normal child a period of vigorous questioning. " Why " and " What " are asked about everything. The inner meaning of this questioning is plainly this, that the child is striving to form his world of concepts into a connected whole within which the same relations between concepts constantly recur. Very interesting is the record of children's questions given by Sully in his *Studies of Childhood*.[1] In some cases children find their way spontaneously to problems over which the acutest brains of theologians and philosophers have puzzled. " Where was I before I was born ? " is a common question as is well known. Sully gives examples of more recondite ones. " When there was no egg, where did the hen come from ? " " If I'd gone upstairs, could God make it that I hadn't ? "

We do not propose to trace subsequent developments in detail. It seems to me plain however that it is the same impulse which ultimately develops into that of scientific enquiry. There is no real reason for drawing a line between the curiosity of the child and that of the scientific enquirer. The one grows into the other. With the great majority of men, as life proceeds, other impulses and needs compete with and nearly altogether oust that of disinterested curiosity ; they are too busy with the support of their own lives to be able to attend systematically to the extension or ordering of knowledge. They rest content with the generalizations embodied in the language of their society, and are only concerned to bring the apparently novel within such generalizations without extending them. A certain number however have the opportunity and the inclination for theoretical pursuits. If we look at the motive of these men, we shall, I think, see it is still for the most part the impulse to achieve the feeling of

[1] See pp. 75–90, 103, and 455–60.

power by ordering the manifold universe into connected
wholes. Darwin will afford us a good example. Darwin
undoubtedly started his enquiry under the influence of
Lyell's *Principles of Geology*. Lyell had argued with
success against catastrophic accounts of the geological
history of the world and in favour of present conditions
having been brought about by the accumulation, over
very long periods of time, of small changes similar to those
now to be observed in operation. In facing the problem
of the origin of species Darwin started with a desire to
find an account which would use only known data and
discard special creations, which could not be represented
in terms of known experience. The difficult problem was
as to " how ", and all his labour of research was devoted
to finding something to bridge the gap between the known
principles of experience and the facts to be accounted for,
those of the difference of species. It is in this search,
be it observed, that mental originativeness is shown.
The struggle for existence and survival of the fittest is
observed on a fragmentary scale operating in the present
world. Thought of as operating throughout biological
history and on a scale sufficient to bring about the selection of organisms and the difference of species, it is a
conception extended so immensely beyond the observed
facts suggesting it as to be rightly called an origination.
In essence however the mental operation is only a higher
form of that which Hobhouse has noted in the adaptation
of tools by monkeys, and called " Analogical extension ",[1]
or the similar process in human thought which Spearman called the " eduction of a correlate ".[2] It was by
using these means that Darwin strove to make the biological history of the world " intelligible ". We see the
same impulse towards unification at work in the laying
down of the principle of the conservation of energy by
Joule and Mayer. " There is little doubt ", writes Ward,

---

[1] Hobhouse, *Mind in Evolution*, 277, 305.
[2] Spearman, *Nature of Intelligence and Principles of Cognition*,
chap. VII.

" that both men first conceived the general truth and then set about—the one by experiments, the other by computations from ascertained physical constants—to verify what they had thus conceived." And the following is quoted from a letter of Mayer : " I discovered the new theory for the sufficient reason that I vividly felt the need of it."[1] The principle of the conservation of energy is indeed only another form given to the law of causality ; and this latter is essentially a demand that the universe, in spite of its apparent qualitative diversity, shall yet be ultimately a quantitative unity, in regard to which predictions can in theory be made with absolute certainty, and in which there do not occur either creations *e nihilo* or annihilations, which would destroy that unity and render any connected account of it impossible.[2] It is this view of the impulse to science, i.e. that it springs from a will to power, which is something which Nietzsche was never tired of repeating.[3] We must however admit that this will to power does not exhaustively describe the motives present in scientific enquiry. There are two other motives present, which must be allowed for. In the first place of course science is also ascertainment of fact. In giving the mind over to the objective facts there is, or may be, more enjoyment of the richness and diversity of the actual world than there is in the tracing of mere law and uniformity. The more knowledge of facts, the fuller seems the mental life. James writes of this spirit, that " it prefers any amount of incoherence, abruptness, and fragmentariness (so long as the literal details of the separate facts are saved) to an abstract way of conceiving

---

[1] Ward, *Naturalism and Agnosticism*, I, 174–5.
[2] How far recent physical theories affect this view of the universe it is not our place to enquire, occupied as we are with the psychological view of the matter. But it certainly seems a fact that the quantum theory, with its view of the discontinuity of the physical universe, has been received generally with a certain dismay or puzzlement. It is not *welcomed*. I happen at the moment to notice a statement in the leading article in *Nature* (22.9.28), to the effect that in the long contest between continuity and discontinuity in the history of science, " continuity will win in the end."
[3] See Nietzsche, *Will to Power*, Vol. II, 20–38.

things, that while it simplifies them, dissolves away at the same time their concrete fulness ".[1] Yet of this enjoy-ment of the concrete fulness of the world we may say that it is hardly the spirit of science. It is rather that of the artist. Secondly, science is also faithfulness to fact. In giving oneself to the ascertainment of fact there is also operative a spirit, as it were, of humility. The facts must be accorded their own rights and we must not force them into our own patterns. The pursuit of pure truth may be thus felt by the agent as a sort of self-giving. It is this feeling which Huxley tried to express when he said that he who would enter the kingdom of science must enter as a little child. Yet, allowing for the above, I think we must still hold that the main motive to science does con-sist in the will to order the objective world by means of thought and make it intelligible. It is this that yields the driving force, whereas respect for facts acts rather as a regulating motive, which prevents an excessive influence of the will to power. No one, however disinterested an enquirer, collects facts aimlessly without any attempted classification of them into uniformities. It would of course be impossible to attempt this. What such an enquirer may do is to rest content with the categories with which current language provides him, without any attempt to extend or alter them. But I should doubt if such mere collection of facts has been common. Darwin was himself one of the most conscientious observers of facts ever known, but there can be no doubt of the motive by which he was impelled.

We can now give a résumé, from the point of view of feeling, of our treatment of the intellectual impulse. There is a normal tendency of the mind, starting from a moment of surprise and non-adaptation in face of a presented object, to move towards clearness and certainty of knowledge, in which its feeling of power is increased. The first stage, that of non-adaptation, cannot be de-

---

[1] Essay on " Sentiment of Rationality " in *The Will to Believe*, 66.

scribed as definitely unpleasant. There is in it rather a stimulus to the activity of the mind ; it is exciting and vivifies the mind. If the feeling of uncertainty continues and no progress is made towards reducing the object to something comprehended, tension may increase and a feeling of impotence and bewilderment may arise, which will be unpleasant. The unpleasure results from the fact that the existing impulse towards adequate cognition has been impeded from progressing towards its end. The existence of the effort is not due to unpleasure having occurred first, and it is not in essence an attempt to get rid of unpleasure. If this were the case, the impulse would be satisfied by the reaching of a condition of indifference or blankness, whereas the end to be attained is rather the heightened consciousness going with the sense of mastery. This feeling can only be attained if there is a movement, and its progress is to some extent gradual. If on the one hand the mind remained in a primitive state of passive receptivity before objects, or if on the other hand a complete understanding existed from the first, without the possibility of ignorance being even imagined, in neither case (assuming their possibility) would the mind fulfil its nature. It is in the movement from the first shock of non-adaptation to the sense of achieved mastery that the inborn nature of the mind is realized ; and this process will be accompanied by pleasure, in so far as it proceeds without undue impediment. There is a possible moment of success in which the pleasure attains its maximum. Thereafter the object, or whole including relations between objects, which is considered to be understood and classified, becomes familiar, and with familiarity any object or idea tends to lose its pleasureableness. To the active mind however it may still appear as a stepping-stone to wider generalizations. As Ward says, when a common principle has been discerned among apparently disconnected particulars, they become as one, " and we seem at once to have at our disposal resources for the command of an enlarged field and the detection of new resem-

I

blances ".[1] It need hardly be said that very few workers in any field of science are likely to be able to make many such original steps. The majority will be limited to rehearsing the steps by which, through the contributions of many workers, the organized body of a science has been built up. But in so doing they are able in some degree to recapture for themselves the thrill of satisfaction which original discovery must have brought. In the course of any scientific enquiry or study there will no doubt often be a hold-up of progress owing to unresolved contradictions or difficulties of comprehension ; and such periods will be relatively unpleasant. There will also be many activities of a subsidiary kind necessary for the prosecution of the main work, but not concerned directly with it, during which pleasure will relatively be less. There must therefore be ups and downs, and variations of feeling. But according as the process is felt to proceed successfully and to involve attainment (if only partial), so the sense of power will increase, and with it pleasure. It is not to be supposed, therefore, that the effective motive is to attain an end state conceived as pleasant. The end state given all at once would be valueless. The only way in which we can conceive of it as giving pleasure in such a case is because after attainment we can imagine ourselves looking back on a pre-existing stage of ignorance and rehearsing again the rise from this to complete knowledge. It is this feeling which Lessing expressed in his often-quoted statement : " Did the Almighty holding in his right hand ' Truth ' and in his left ' Search after Truth ' deign to tender me the one I might prefer ; in all humility, but without hesitation, I should request ' Search after Truth.' "[2] Stevenson too has said : " To travel hopefully is better than to arrive ". Yet in form perhaps these statements contain a certain exaggeration. Relative and partial success at least must be aimed at and con-

---

[1] Ward, *Psychological Principles*, 258.
[2] Quoted by Sir W. Hamilton, *Metaphysics*, I, 13, who gives other illustrations.

sidered possible, or there would be no incentive for the search. A search which appeared certain to be entirely barren and fruitless would never be undertaken. A search means a will to success, and it is not possible at the same time to desire and not to desire success. The state of mind of such an enquirer should therefore logically be one in which endeavour is made to achieve a sustained and regular progress, marked by points of partial success ; and each partial success would appear as a stage opening up further vistas of effort after completeness of knowledge.

CHAPTER IV

THE IMPULSE TO POWER

THE existence of an instinct of self-assertion has been generally recognized of late, and it has often been considered the most important of the human instincts. It seems to me hardly possible to discuss its ultimate nature at all adequately, without at least touching on the question of the consciousness of self, with which it must be closely connected. It is possible to hold, as a fact of psychological observation, that there is a sense of self involved in all perception, inasmuch as the object must always appear as something " given " or " imposed ", i.e. as something foreign to or independent of a perceiving subject; and that thus all conscious experience occurs in the form " subject-perceiving-object ". It would carry us unnecessarily far if we endeavoured to discuss this question at all fully. There must however in any case, so it seems to me, be some sense of self as soon as any living being, in order to fulfil an instinctive impulse arising from its own nature, is aware that it is necessary to effect an alteration in an object presented to it. In such a case the object appears as presenting a persisting inertia, which has to be altered by the only means which the conscious mind can directly control, i.e. by bodily movements. The bodily movements must conform to the object. And we can hardly doubt therefore that when an object presents itself as " something to be altered from what it is ", there is in a rudimentary form the awareness of a distinction between the self and a not-self. A simple case is that of the living being moving towards food. The impulse arising from hunger sensation is something that qualifies the self, that belongs to the subjective side of experience, as contrasted with the food-object, which, in order that the hunger arising may be satisfied, has to be manipulated and altered. The food, when perceived, is an object which persists as it is, and to which the movements have to be adapted, in order to effect that alteration in it which leads to the satisfaction of hunger.

It is perhaps possible that a complete form of self-consciousness could arise through the mere fact of adaptation to the external forces of inanimate nature. If we can assume a gradual increase of intellectual power, there would go with it the capacity to hold a given object before the mind and to pursue its attainment during a period of time by varied means and against various obstacles. In such case there might develop with increasing clearness an awareness of a distinction between the object to be obtained and incidental obstacles on the one hand, and the striving self with its hunger impulse on the other. But it is hardly possible to judge of this possibility, as no living being exists in isolation from other living beings. Self-consciousness in its more complete form, as we know it, appears to arise as the result of relations to other living beings. Relations of co-operation may be supposed to play some part. In any form of co-operative work, including that of male and female in the care and rearing of the offspring, there must be some awareness on the part of the agent of himself in relation to outside agents other than and yet similar to himself; for all his activities have to be adjusted to the resembling and yet different activities of those others. It is however from relations of opposition that self-consciousness arises in that clearer and more definite form which leads to the sense of power; and it is that with which we are concerned here. Suppose another animal seizes the food at the same time as the first, the series of movements leading to food absorption is interrupted. The first animal will for a moment still endeavour to get the food; and then finding itself prevented, by an easy transition turns on the rival, and a combat ensues in which each,

using its body in the way to which the inherited structure
adapts it, endeavours to crush the opposition of the other.
In the moment of such conflict there is, as it appears to
me, an immediate awareness of force meeting opposing
force. The one agent is aware of his own movements
as directly expressing his mental urge, that towards
hunger satisfaction. The experience is that of impulse
passing into movement; and roughly speaking, the
energy of the movement is proportionate to the intensity
of the mental urge ; for the more violent hunger passes
into the more violent movement, first of grasping and then
of fighting.[1] But the movements of the opponent are
understood at once as expressing an urge similar to that
of the agent's own. In order to give an adequate account
of this point it is necessary to go back to the primitive
facts of the cognitive apprehension of the external world.
From the first a factor which has been effective in helping
to build up our ideas of a world of separate things independent of us has been what has been called a " projection of self ".[2] In the first place we attribute implicitly
to an object, in so far as it gives us a cue by its separate-
ness from other objects, a persisting identity with itself
in the intervals between our different perceptions, an
identity similar to that of which we are aware in our own
bodily self. In the second place, again in so far as the
object itself gives some sort of initial cue, e.g. by its movement as a whole, the primitive mind attributes implicitly
to the persisting object something of the same sort of
inner life as that which it experiences itself. That which
prevents our movement appears to us to do so in
virtue of the same sort of conative effort of which we are

---

[1] It is difficult to give an account which altogether avoids trespass-
ing on disputed questions. I do not think the mode of expression in
the text is faulty, even if we have to admit that no consciousness at all
accompanies the efferent nervous discharge, i.e. that from the motor
cells to the muscles. It would still be the case that the more intense
hunger impulse (a fact of which the agent is directly aware) is followed
by movement which yields muscle and joint sensations of proportionately greater intensity.
[2] See Ward, *Psychological Principles*, 165–6, and Stout, *Groundwork
of Psychology*, 96–100.

conscious ourselves; the experience of resisted effort is interpreted as implying something which exerts a counter-effort. And there is also attributed to the object something of the same organic unity as that in ourselves; it appears as having a wholeness of existence in itself, a sympathy between its various parts. It is only carrying the same process a stage further when the primitive mind explicitly personifies objects, e.g. when the child punishes a chair for being naughty or when the savage treats trees, rivers, rocks, etc., as having a life similar to his own. But this explicit anthropomorphism is not necessary, though it often occurs. Speaking generally, the distinction between the inanimate external to us and the animate external to us is very early made. This distinction is principally based on the differing form of the movements of animate and inanimate, a fact which has been emphasized by the school of "form psychology". The contact with the opponent, in the particular case before us, not only prevents the intended movement of the agent. But also the visual sensations and the tactual sensations (given by bodily contact), due to the movements of the opponent, are identical or closely similar in form and tempo with the sequence of joint and muscle sensations and the visual sensations, due to the agent's own movements, a form which is quite different to that of the movement of the inanimate. Each series of sensations (visual and kinæsthetic on the one hand, visual and tactual on the other) has the same temporal relations constituting its form, i.e. one in which in the particular case before us would be described by such terms as "jerky", "violent", or "excited". It is in such a way that Koffka surmises there may be a direct "understanding" by an onlooker of the meaning of the expressive movements of another, even by animals or infants.[1] Given the primitive tendency to projection of self, it is then very easy for the agent to fill out the movements of the opponent (as perceived by sight and

[1] Koffka, *Growth of the Mind*, 115–18 and 133–6.

touch) with the same sort of emotions and impulses as he experiences in himself. This inference need not be explicitly made. But he will behave on the basis of the supposition that what is impeding him is the striving of another self, even though he may not be able to formulate the belief. In the course of the struggle then the agent will either find himself constraining and bending to his will the opposing effort of his adversary, or he will find the adverse self constraining him. In the first case there will be awareness of a perceptual situation, to be described as " superior power " or " dominance "; in the latter to be described as " inferior power ", or " subjection ", accompanied most likely by physical pain. In the former case the cognitive apprehension of the situation will be accompanied by a subjective state of feeling which will be pleasant, in the latter it will be unpleasant, and in both cases there will be, as it were, a reverberation over the whole conscious life. The successful affirmation of the self as against opposing force seems to raise the level of all the conscious processes, so that life seems an intenser and more valuable thing. There is a rebound from the incipient depression which was threatened when defeat was possible (it being assumed that the struggle was in some degree a close one). An animal in such circumstances, or a human being who has not reached the stage of deliberate self-control, shows this enhancement in various ways such as prancing, strutting, shouting with joy, etc. The defeated one on the other hand slinks away showing his depression in all his gestures or attitudes, a depression which may be partly due to the fact of unsuccessful self-assertion against the adversary, and partly also to the mere fact that physical suffering has been inflicted which could not be resisted.

The explanation, or interpretation, of these phenomena which we endeavour to give is on the following lines. In all the effort of any living being to maintain its bodily life with the functions pertaining thereto there is contained some sort of self-affirmation. The effort of life, as we have

described it in dealing with sensory pleasure and unpleasure, is one to maintain the course of certain sensations,
those going with the bodily processes. There is intimately
bound up with the existence of these sensations a self
as a centre of the sensations and a uniting bond between
them. The effort, so I would affirm, is always to prolong
into the future this unit of consciousness which, however
closely bound up with the bodily sensations, is not identical
with them, and to which the bodily sensations are capable
of becoming objects. The mind indeed of its own nature
seems always to live a forward-looking existence. It is
essentially an effort to self-prolongation into the future.
If life from the biological point of view consists in the
maintenance of a given form, it does not seem unreasonable to suppose that there is a consciousness bound up
with that form, which is also maintained. When this
conscious centre successfully maintains itself in its functions as against any difficulty or obstruction, there must,
we may assume, be a rudimentary form of heightened
self-feeling or elation. But this elation will only be
evanescent and will give no outward sign of its existence
until in the course of development two factors appear :
(1) There must be the capacity to realize with some distinctness the nature of the resistant force which is overcome. The self cannot be felt as affirmed except relatively
to opposing force, and most clearly in relation to the
opposition of another self. No marked degree of elation
will be felt until it is realized more or less clearly that
dominance has been exercised over some other self.
(2) There must be the capacity to retain some abiding
memory of the success (or defeat), which thus is able to
bring about a more or less enduring mood of elation (or
depression). No doubt the first result of success in any
contest against opposition may be only a consciousness
of freedom from the constraint exercised by the adversary.
But this in itself is only negative, due to the effects of
contrast, and will not last for long. That which was
originally sought was the maintenance of the conscious

life, the prevention of its depression to a lower level; but that which is attained in the course of the effort may be the raising of it to a higher level. Everyone knows how in practical life it is difficult to draw the line between self-defence and aggression. In any contest, in order to protect oneself, it is necessary to initiate some sort of counter-attack and to go beyond merely meeting the moves of the adversary as they are made; and it is thus that self-defence passes by insensible gradations in the course of a struggle into the effort to crush the adversary. In the same way during the course of the contest the will to maintenance of the conscious life can pass by insensible gradations into the will for its enhancement. But of course a further step is involved if, in the absence of any contest and when unprovoked, the living being goes out with apparent spontaneity to aim at dominance over others and the enhancement of self-feeling going therewith. It would be going too far to say that life has from the first striven directly towards its own enhancement, that there has always existed " Life's incessant aspiration to higher organization, wider and deeper self-consciousness ".[1] It would be more correct, I think, to suppose that a process of development takes place in the following way. Suppose that a living being, which has once, or oftener, experienced the rebound of elation coming with success after a difficult struggle, finds itself with a certain amount of superfluous energy after the ordinary vital needs have been satisfied. Another living being appears of the same kind as that against which the previous contest took place, or else a situation similar to that of the previous struggle recurs. There may then be a suggestion (faint perhaps) of possible contest, the other living being may appear as a rival offering a potential challenge, or the situation may present a suggestion as of something to be overcome. This suggestion will then lead to a sort of inner repetition or rehearsal of the previous series of mental events, in which that portion of

---

[1] Bernard Shaw, *Man and Superman*, Act III.

the series which consisted in the will to dominance will be
magnified, as it were, by the existing store of superfluous
mental energy. The suggestion of a contest, that is to
say, will call out a needlessly violent reaction, which will
take the form of a rebound and effort towards that
experience of dominance which occurred before in the
same connection. Thus there will tend to come into
existence a will which aims directly and consciously
at power ; and a living being endowed with sufficient
memory and intellectual capacity will always be capable
of thus making power an end. But this must not be described as the emergence of a new motive to action. It is
only the self-assertion already latent in the self-preserving
acts of every living being, which has now become intensified and more conscious of itself. In speaking of the will
to power we must be understood to mean that the end
sought is the cognitive situation of " dominance ", with
the accompanying feeling of elation. We do not necessarily imply that the feeling can be made an end in itself.
As regards the feeling of elation itself, I do not see how it
can be analysed further than in the description we have
already given. It includes a heightened consciousness of
self, but also something more, the feeling of the triumphant self, which results in a radiation over the whole
mental life, raising it to a higher level of energy and intensity. Enhanced self-consciousness is yielded in the fact
of struggle, not necessarily of victory. In the awareness
of power superior to one's own and contrasted with it,
the self may be felt as intensely as when there is awareness
of inferior power which is being overcome. Doubtless
there is a value to be ascribed to the enhancement of self-
consciousness resulting from unsuccessful struggle. It is
in respect of its increased self-consciousness that we
attribute a greater value to the life of a man than to that
of a tortoise. But this is another matter into which we
may hope to go later.

As stated above, it is not easy to be sure at what point
in development dominance or victory in combat begins

to be sought as an end, beyond the object in dispute, whatever it may be, food or a mate or something else. But certainly the fact is to be observed among many of the higher animals. The institution of leadership exists in the herds of many gregarious species. Leadership on the part of the male in many cases carries with it the possession of a band of females with opportunities of sexual gratification ; and this no doubt affords the motive for a good deal of fighting between males. But we also see the signs of satisfaction in mere dominance. Hudson has written as follows of the packs of semi-wild dogs kept on the cattle-breeding establishments in South America : " From the foremost in strength down to the weakest there is a gradation of authority ; each one knows just how far he can go, which companion he can bully when in a bad temper or wishes to assert himself, and to which he must humbly yield in his turn ".[1] The leader, who has won his position in combat, acquires a lasting sentiment of dominance so long as he remains undefeated, while the others have a lasting sentiment of subjection in relation to him. The existence of a permanent relationship of mutual authority and subjection can also be observed in bands of anthropoid apes. The leader acquires his position by fighting other males and thereafter shows his sense of his position by the supervision and care which he exercises over them in various ways. The dependence of the others on the leader is shown if he is shot ; they are for a moment rigid with terror and bewilderment and then flee wildly in all directions.[2] The sense of injured pride can also be illustrated by the many stories told of monkeys and elephants, who have remembered an injury for lengthy periods and eventually " got even with " the author of it by inflicting some damage on him.[3] The satisfaction of mere overcoming can be observed in the domestic dog.

[1] Hudson, *Naturalist in La Plata*, 337.
[2] See description by Pechuel Lœsche in Brehm's *Tierleben* (1920), *Säugetiere*, Vol. 4, 507.
[3] Thus see the story of revenge by a baboon, quoted by Darwin, *Descent of Man*, 105.

He enjoys the mock combat of pulling with any object, of no value in itself, against some person as an opponent, and aims keenly at success. The attraction of " forbidden fruit " also plainly exists. He likes sometimes to steal the cat's dinner though he has refused his own ; there being a suggestion in this of the results of successful combat.

In the foregoing we have taken physical combat as the occasion which most clearly calls out the will to power, as it is perhaps also the earliest. But there are other forms of resistance by which it is called out, and there are ways by which power can be exercised other than by physical force. In human societies compulsion is as a rule exercised by means of the suggestion of physical force in the background, which can be employed if necessary, as indeed is the case in some of the animal societies which we have mentioned. In human societies there is also the power of wealth, by means of which constraint can be exercised on others by awarding or withholding the means of subsistence. Wealth is sought largely for the sense of power which it gives. There is also the authority often accorded by tradition to certain ranks, names, or positions, which cause them to be objects of desire. We also have the many forms of emulation and competition, other than by physical combat. The satisfaction given by success in emulative competition with others arises, so we may believe, in the following way. When some valuable object, such as food, is in dispute, the possession of it may be decided by other qualities as well as mere physical strength, for example, superior speed, skill, cunning, or far-sightedness. Possibly even in the animal world there may be some satisfaction in getting the better of an adversary by these qualities, apart from the pleasure of getting the valuable object itself. This feeling becomes intensified in man ; and an important development is due to the fact that qualities can now be abstracted in thought and named, so that it is possible for sentiments of value to grow up round the ideas of such qualities as lead to success in life. If a man measures himself against others in respect of physical speed or skill, or in various forms of intellectual capacity such as memory or far-sightedness, and can reckon himself as superior, his self-feeling is enhanced ; he has a feeling of pride. When a sentiment of self has been acquired, i.e. as soon as a man comes to have some idea of himself as an abiding personality with a certain character, such qualities come to be regarded as valuable elements of this character in themselves and apart from their utility. Hence a large part of the pleasure given by success in the serious competitions of life, e.g. that for the attainment of wealth in business, and, I suppose, the whole of the pleasure yielded by success in emulative sports and games.

There is another form of self-assertive pride, it would seem, which consists in the display before onlookers of valuable qualities and in making an impression on them. In its most developed form this is the love of approbation and fame. As it has been supposed that self-display, particularly by the male animal at the mating season, is the earliest form in which the impulse of self-feeling is shown, it may be worth while to devote a little attention to this point.[1] There can be little doubt, I imagine, that much of the behaviour of animals at the courting season is the result of nothing but an overflow of exuberant energy. At this period there is a rising tide of physical excitement, and it is natural that it should show itself in the behaviour of the animal. Groos describes how at the mating season in certain species of birds (storks and birds of prey) both male and female take part in wonderful flying performances, circling up into the sky and shooting down again with closed wings and so on.[2] Here there can be no question of the male showing off before the female ; the actions must be those of sheer exuberance of spirits. We find moreover it is stated by observers that the

[1] By McDougall, *Introduction to Social Psychology*, 62–6. In his later work, the *Outline of Psychology* (157–8), he attributes more importance in the genesis of self-assertion to combat within the herd.

[2] Groos, *Spiele der Tiere*, 262–3.

so-called courting pose is often that which is assumed
under any strong emotion, such as anger, and it is sometimes displayed by the hen equally with the cock.[1] There
is doubtless a certain joy felt in performing these exercises
owing to the rising tide of physical power ; but there need
be no actual awareness of power exercised on other living
beings. There are however also other species of birds in
which displays are certainly given by the male before the
female. It would probably be right to consider, as
Groos does,[2] that in the course of racial history these
special forms of display have differentiated themselves
from the above-mentioned exuberant movements at the
courting season, though it is certainly difficult to see what
survival advantage to the race or to the individual
could have been yielded by some of the more remarkable
forms of adornment displayed by birds of paradise, peacocks, and other birds. We can however leave the question of biological origins open and look at the facts as
now existing. The most striking instances of display
are probably those given by peacocks and male pheasants.
The gorgeous crests and tails are displayed before the
female clearly in such a way as best to be seen by her, as
Darwin has carefully shown in detail.[3] The male also
can be seen to be observing the effect produced on the
female ; he is as a rule plainly watching the female before
whom he is displaying, and the Argus pheasant, whose fan
of wing feathers, when raised for display, quite conceals his
own head, is often seen pushing his head through it in
order to watch the female.[4] Groos has given all this a full
treatment, and he is probably right in saying that the male
at these times must have some awareness of the effect
that he is producing on the female, and that there is a form
of self-consciousness present. But it does not follow that
this self-consciousness has the form of self-assertive pride.
The whole display originates under the urge of the sexual

---

[1] See Finn, *Bird Behaviour*, 268 and 300, and Espinas, *Des Sociétés
Animales*, 181.
[2] *Spiele der Tiere*, 267.
[3] Darwin, *Descent of Man*, 603 ff.   [4] Darwin, op. cit., 607.

instinct. In as far as this only is working, we should hardly speak of pride. The courting frame of mind is not in itself one of pride or self-confidence, but rather one of pleading.[1] Until success is attained, a sense of possible failure must always be present in the background. The effect to be produced on the onlooking female is moreover definitely a sexual one, not mere approbation by itself. It is said that the peacock will show off his finery before poultry or even pigs.[2] This we must describe as a playful exercise, due to superfluous energy, of an instinctive tendency for its own sake, though the normal stimulus for its exercise is not present. It may thus contain in a rudimentary form the impulse to attract others and make an impression, apart from any sexual effect. But the facts are rare and the interpretation doubtful. On the whole it seems to me right to conclude that the courting displays of animals are activities subsidiary to sexual ends, and do not include any appreciable element of self-assertion in the form of the impulse to dominate and impress others.

The desire of approbation and fame, properly so called, seems to arise in the following manner. As already mentioned, certain qualities are useful to the possessor because they enable him to maintain his own life and carry out its functions successfully, and in the case of competition with others to secure the object in dispute against them. Hence as soon as a man is capable of forming ideas about himself, they come to be thought of as valuable for their own sake. There is also a certain sense of health and general well-being which is given by the harmonious and easy exercise of such bodily capacities as speed and strength, and at a later stage by exercising intellectual power. This sense of well-being combines with the satisfaction felt in the possession of valuable qualities which

---

[1] Cf. Pycraft, *Courtship of Animals*, 142. " In the case of the warblers the male in these ecstatic moods will commonly hold a leaf or a piece of stick in his beak as if suggesting the work of nest-building and its delightful sequence.'' This or its equivalent is a common phase in other species, he continues.

[2] Darwin, op. cit., 600.

enable one to surpass one's competitors. Thus an inner pride is felt in the possession of these qualities. But this self-esteem is not as a rule a thing we are satisfied with by itself. We tend to ask for confirmation of it by others. The deference which we pay to society and our general sense of dependence on it disposes us to accept in the main the judgment which it passes on our own capacities, as on those of others. It is difficult to feel any decided superiority in any valuable quality unless we have confirmation of the judgment by others. "It is in order to fix and confirm their valuable opinion of themselves, not from any original passion, that men seek the applauses of others."[1] But Hume goes too far in completely denying the existence of any "original passion" for fame. When a man is famous we feel, not only that society has recognized and confirmed his possession of valuable qualities, but also that in some way he has constrained it to do so, by making it pay attention to something forceful and impressive, and that of this the successful man must be to some extent aware. This may go so far that a desire may arise merely to impress society and make oneself well known, apart from any consideration of the means by which this is brought about. This is the desire for mere notoriety. There is thus involved in our ordinary attitude towards the opinion of society both submissive and self-assertive tendencies ; and indeed this is the case with all our relations towards our society, as we shall hope to show in further detail a little further on.

The sense of power with its accompanying elation may be elicited, and may become an end to be attained, in other situations besides those involving relations to other living beings. We have already mentioned the resistance which the inertia of inanimate things offers to actions of living beings as a possible subsidiary occasion for the growth of self-consciousness and the sense of power.

[1] Hume, *Dissertation on the Passions*, Sec. II, 10 (p. 152, Vol. IV, Green and Gross's edition); cf. *Treatise of Human Nature*, Bk. II, Part 1, sec. 11.

K

There can be no doubt that the first impulse of any living being is to treat any opposition as proceeding from a will similar to its own. In the case of other living beings this expectation is confirmed by the intuitive understanding of their movements, as we have already explained. The inert opposition of the inanimate is something quite different and so comes to be treated differently. Nevertheless there is an elation due to successful self-assertion over this inertia, though less intense than that in relation to the animate. Anyone who has cut down a tree with the axe must have known the thrill of power, when as the result of his exertions the tree crashes down, laid in the desired direction. It is as though a tall antagonist had been overthrown. The need for the satisfaction of overcoming may lead to the creation of artificial obstacles, even in the case of an animal. A dog, known to the writer, had once, apparently by accident, rolled his ball into a difficult position behind a piece of furniture and only got it out again after a considerable struggle ; thereafter when no human would play with him, he often rolled the ball into the same position again, plainly moved by the wish to find some sort of challenge or opposition to overcome. Stern says of a child fifteen months old that he would set himself little tasks to accomplish, for example, pushing his roll and butter after one bite on to the top of the table where it was difficult to reach again.[1] There is also a joy in the mere fact of being a cause, of being able to produce results in the external world, which is to be observed both in animals and children. The love of destruction for its own sake by monkeys is well known. Miss Romanes tells a number of stories on this point of the cebus monkey kept by her. " To-day he got hold of a wineglass and an egg cup. The glass he dashed on the floor with all his might and of course broke it. Finding however that the egg cup would not break for being thrown down, he looked round for some hard substance against which to dash it. The post of the brass bedstead appearing

[1] Stern, *Psychology of Early Childhood*, 445.

to be suitable for the purpose, he raised the egg cup high over his head and gave it several hard blows. When it was completely smashed he was quite satisfied."[1] The same sort of impulse is exemplified in children from a very early age. It is possible that the first production of change in external things may occur as the result of accidental movement by the child. But the child soon finds out that, having an impulse for such results again, it is able to realize them by movements of its own body ; the results prefigured in the state of desire or expectation can be brought into objective existence. Hence the consciousness of agency, of being a cause. " Why do all children take such wonderful delight in noise they make themselves ? I believe because their own efforts produce it, and because causality is such a very early feeling. The child beating an enamel tray on a wooden table creates something—something too that can be heard."[2] " Destructive " play occurs earlier in children than " constructive ". The sense of being a cause is very easily and quickly obtained by destroying or throwing down. Children from a very early age delight in tearing up paper, throwing down the brick edifices built for them by others, putting the well-ordered into confusion and so on. Constructive games need more patience, accuracy, and foresight, and so are a somewhat later development. It is not necessary to describe in detail the pleasure taken in such activities as house-building with sand, bricks, etc. In all these we see exemplified the impulse to self-assertion by the means of impressing desired results on the external world.[3]

The last form of the exercise of power which we shall mention is that shown in power over one's own body. Groos has said that the first object in the struggle for mastery is the body, whose subjection is obtained through

[1] Romanes, *Animal Intelligence*, 484.
[2] Stern, *Psychology of Early Childhood*, 130.
[3] Detailed descriptions are given by Stern, *Psychology of Early Childhood*, 310–15; Groos, *Spiele der Menschen*, 118–23, amongst others.

experimentation and plays of movement.[1] As we have
remarked in dealing with combat, the bodily movements
are the way in which the will to self-maintenance must
primarily express itself, there being no other means by
which ordinarily effects can be produced on the external
world.   In this respect the sensations of movement are
treated as appertaining to the subjective side of experience over against the obstacle offered by outside resistance.
With all the higher animals however there is a stage of
life at which the power to use the body in order to bring
about change in some needed direction is imperfect.
In particular the control and exercise of the chief racial
movements, e.g. walking, are only gradually acquired.
The gradual learning by the child of these movements
appears undoubtedly to be accompanied by the sense of
mastery, as of difficulties surmounted and of a new experience created, just in the same way as the adult has a sense
of increased power when he learns some new bodily
exercise, such as skating, dancing, bicycling.   " It is well
established ", writes Froebel,[2] " that walking, and especially the first walking, gives joy to the child purely as a
manifestation of power, though there is certainly soon
added to this other joy-creating perceptions, in being
able to come to something and reach something."   The
germ of power consciousness, which is contained herein,
can be much increased by the contrast felt between
doing things alone and under compulsion or with help ;
since at so many points the child has to rely on grown-up
help, he is all the more consumed with desire to be able
to do without that help whenever he possibly can.   " Do
it by myself, walk by myself, build by myself, is his cry at
every turn ".[3]   There is also a constant desire to show off
before others and obtain their applause ; the pride of
success requires confirmation by the applause of an
audience.   In adult life there is a certain sense of power

---

[1] Groos, *Spiele der Tiere*, 296.
[2] Quoted by Groos, *Spiele der Menschen*, 100.
[3] Stern, *Psychology of Early Childhood*, 481.

going with bodily vigour and health, which contributes to the total state of feeling due to bodily well-being. In waking life a pull of gravity is always being exercised on the body, and this is counteracted by the constant tonic contraction of certain muscles; the head is kept upright by the neck muscles, the lower jaw is kept up against the upper by its own muscles, and the eyelids are kept raised.[1] In full wakefulness and health these muscular contractions are easily maintained against the gravitational pull and a sense of lightness and power is thus yielded; whereas when we are tired and weak, the head falls about, the lower jaw drops, and the eyelids droop, with the result that there is a bodily consciousness of heaviness and impotence. As Souriau and Groos[2] have well pointed out the pleasures of rapid movement are largely due to the same sort of cause. Our ordinary movements, and particularly our attempts to move fast, are always retarded by the pull of gravitation together with the friction of the ground surface. Any rapid gliding movement, in which these are for the time being annulled, gives us a delightful impression of freedom and power. Swinging, sailing, skating, tobogganing, motoring, are all examples of this. It is not so much the overcoming of gravitational force, so much as that of friction, which gives us the impression of freedom. For, as Groos remarks, there is nothing more exhilarating than the downward rush of tobogganing, in which we do not resist, but give full play to, the effects of gravitation. What we are freed from in these cases is that dependence on the ground surface and need of adjustment to it which exercise so constant a retardation and compulsion over all our movements. Indeed there is a peculiar pleasure in any frictionless movement even if not particularly rapid; e.g. any form of gliding or floating, provided of course the disturbance of equilibrium is not extreme. There are other factors of a sensory character in the pleasure of

[1] See Höffding, *Outlines of Psychology*, 226.
[2] See Groos, *Spiele der Tiere*, 301 and 302.

rapid movement which contribute to make it one of the intensest of human pleasures : in the first place, as I think, an effect of a peculiar intoxicating character, either exciting or soothing, probably due to the action of the labyrinthine apparatus ; in the second place, the stimulating effect on the organism generally produced by the unusually rapid change in the visual appearance of objects.   But the sense of power is also a factor.

Yet I do not think that in these experiences generally we shall find an important original source of the sense of power in human beings.   There can only be a rudimentary consciousness of self involved in the learning of movements by the child, that is to say if they are regarded by themselves apart from an audience.   The body can hardly be treated as something external so as to yield a consciousness of self-hood over against it.   In adult life the pleasure of mastering new forms of bodily exercise is very closely bound up with our relations to our fellows.   The exercises are of the sort which we have seen others perform and we always, I think, ask for some appreciation from others. There is a sense of power no doubt in rapid and easy movement, but only in any marked form, I imagine, for those who in other ways, chiefly through the different forms of contact with other living beings in social life, have acquired a developed self-consciousness.   As we humans watch an eagle wheeling high up in the air with outstretched wings, seeming to surge forward, as it were, by the effortless exercise of some inner force, it gives us an indescribable impression of majesty and power. " Sailing with supreme dominion ", the poet describes it. But we have no assurance that we are justified in reading these feelings of ours into the eagle itself, even in its first performances ; for its self-consciousness, so far as we know, must be of a very rudimentary character.

An important point which we must note with regard to the consciousness of power is that it enters as an element giving additional pleasure and value into the exercise of a number of other instincts.   We have already remarked this in regard to the acquisition of a movement, such as walking, and have also shown in detail how it gives the chief element of value found in the acquisition of knowledge. Let us also take the instinct of construction, so-called. Many species of animals show instincts leading to the construction of shelters of various sorts for themselves and for their offspring. These instincts are in their origin subsidiary to the more general impulses which aim at the protection of the body from injury and at protection of the young. We must leave the question of their precise origin doubtful, i.e. whether it is possible to regard such tendencies to construction as originating as accidental variations, or whether there was some sort of purpose of protection in them from the start. In any case the tendency to the construction of specific sorts of shelter has certainly become fixed by heredity, and so the instinct is exercised in captivity even when useless. The bird builds nests in captivity, the captive beaver collects twigs and straws and tries to build.[1] Chimpanzees in captivity show tendencies to the construction of nests, which however rarely reach completion.[2] It is possible that man may have inherited some rudimentary tendency towards shelter building from his ape-like ancestors. But it is plain that all such tendencies are towards the construction of certain specific forms of shelter and could not of themselves lead to the generalized constructiveness which we find in man. It must surely be evident that, for man as we know him now, the exercise of the constructive impulse derives all its pleasurableness and value from the enhancement of self-feeling, i.e. because in building up something a man feels that he has impressed himself and his plans on the external world. Not that the mere fact of production of change will continue to satisfy for long, apart from any question of a further value in the object produced. Only young children are satisfied with the causation of aimless change. In later life we

---

[1] Schneider, *Der Tierische Wille*, 217.
[2] Köhler, *The Mentality of Apes*, 93-4.

demand that the work shall have some further effectiveness, particularly in the form of the impression produced on other persons, whether as giving them pleasure, or exercising on them some other dominant effect.

We shall find the same sort of result if we look at the acquisitive instinct. There is an instinctive impulse to hoard, which derives its origin from the need of nutrition. There are a number of animals, squirrels, rats, voles, and others, which in the presence of eatable objects, more than can be consumed at the moment, carry them away and store them for the future. This instinct must have been extremely valuable for the survival of those species in which it was developed. It is often carried out in captivity in a remarkably mechanical manner. There are accounts given of squirrels which in captivity have gone through a sort of imitation of all the movements of burying a nut on a blanket or carpet, in fact of course leaving it quite uncovered.[1] Primarily this instinct must have been highly specialized, only coming into exercise in the presence of the specific object which serves as food for that species, e.g. a nut or grain of wheat. We may assume that it owes its origin to a certain unwillingness to be parted from an object, which, though it cannot at once be eaten, yet remains an object of interest to the animal, as being its ordinary food. Certainly there is a remarkable extension of this impulse to be found in some species. Some birds such as jackdaws will, as is well known, carry away and store up all sorts of bright and shining objects, and rats have been known to do the same. Presumably the explanation of these actions is that the bright objects are pleasing to the animal because of the satisfaction which they give to a craving for sensory stimulation, and hence there is a certain effort to maintain contact with the articles. We should hardly be justified in calling this a general instinct of acquisitiveness. The love of property seems to have another possible source in the

---

[1] James, *Principles of Psychology*, II, 400, quoting Schmidt; and Koffka, *Growth of the Mind*, 88-9.

animal world. We find in a great many species of animals that claim is made to the exclusive possession of a certain territory, even if it be limited only to a special lair, nest, or den. It is obvious that this grows out of the need of the animal to protect its own bodily life from injury; the lair is something which contributes to its bodily well-being. There are claims also to more extended property in land. A pack of wolves is said to maintain exclusive possession of a certain territory as a hunting district, and battles for feeding grounds have been witnessed between troops of baboons and others of the monkey tribes.[1] The way in which the domestic dog resents intrusion on his own premises is well known. All these impulses must be in origin subsidiary to the impulse to preserve life by nutrition; they spring from the need of protecting a source of food supply. When we turn to human beings, we find that food supplies are stored, but we need not appeal to an instinct unconscious of its own meaning in order to explain this. It is done with conscious foresight as provision for future needs. It is however claimed that an instinct of acquisitiveness is shown where there is the tendency to collect objects which could not be useful, or which there is no intention to use. Thus the tendency to collect something, stamps, eggs, etc., is said to be nearly universal among children. Statistics have shown that only a small proportion of those questioned had never collected anything.[2] Excessive development of this instinct is alleged to be exemplified in the miser who hoards without any intention of using his wealth; and pathological forms of this are recorded in such cases as that quoted by James, of a man whose rooms after his death were found crammed with old newspapers, wrapping paper, worn-out umbrellas, canes, pieces of common wire, cast-off clothing, etc. etc. Kleptomania is also brought forward as a pathological excess of the acquisitive instinct. It is perhaps possible that man may have derived from

---

[1] See Carveth Read, *Origin of Man*, 44 and 56–9.
[2] James, *Principles of Psychology*, II, 423.

pre-human ancestors some rudimentary tendency to form a hoard, originally of food, and afterwards of other useful objects ; but it seems somewhat doubtful, as the anthropoid apes are said not to hoard. The satisfaction which human beings take in the accumulation or possession of property of any sort can be accounted for as follows, I think. In the first place we must admit the existence of an innate need for the exclusive possession of a certain territory, whether limited or wide. The sense of a " home " is something very fundamental in our nature, as closely connected with preservation both of self and offspring. Beyond this, where pleasure is found in the acquisition and exclusive possession of objects or property with no prevision of use in the future, there would appear to be two factors at work : (1) Money, or other articles which, even if not valuable in the ordinary sense of the word, yet present themselves as possibly usable in the future, are collected and hoarded with some idea, more or less definite, of future use. A man may then come to regard his accumulation as a sort of permanent reserve, affording the possibility of numberless gratifications in the future, amongst them perhaps the exercise of power over others. He continues to think of the indefinite possibilities bound up with the possession of stores of money or other articles, and may eventually come to prefer the pleasure of this " free ideal activity ", as Stout terms it, to the gratifications that would be attained by actual use.[1] The main reason for this preference is that, in the spending or use, the gratification appears as temporary ; what is once spent is gone for ever ; whereas the gloating over the possibilities of the store is something which can be indefinitely repeated without being used up. In this form of the value ascribed to an accumulated hoard I do not think the sense of power is an essential factor. The possession of a reserve does yield a certain feeling of security and strength. But power is only one of the desirable

---

[1] See Stout, *Analytic Psychology*, II, 90, who gives this line of a rgument.

objects which can be imagined as obtainable by the use or spending of the store. (2) The possession of a store of articles or that of a large amount of property (e.g. in land) means that the self has a wide area over which it exercises control. It can control and dominate a certain section of the outside world. Self-feeling is therefore heightened by the thought of the extended power of the self. But it will not reach any very high degree, unless the possessions are such as in themselves to yield some feeling of value. Either they are rare and difficult to get, in which case their possession symbolizes the valuable qualities (such as strength or some form of skill) which have had to be shown in order to obtain them, or else they are valuable only because sought by other people as well, in which case one's own possession of them signifies the fact that in some way one has surpassed, or got the better of, those others. As a rule both these factors are operative as regards collections. The articles collected have a certain initial rarity ; and also others compete in trying to get them. When once a fashion has been started in collecting certain articles (e.g. stamps) the intrinsic interest of the articles is of little importance. The main value of the collection for the possessor consists in the fact of having been able to compete successfully with others for what is rare, and in being able to exhibit before others the collection which signifies this fact.

On the whole therefore I think that the love of acquisition and property-possessing by men can be sufficiently accounted for without recourse being had to any special instinct. In the account as we have sketched it the love of power is an important element. It would not be difficult to show how the will to power forms at least an important element in other instinctive tendencies of men, such as the hunting impulse, and combativeness or pugnacity. In these instances the part it plays is obvious and need not be insisted on in detail.

We have thus reviewed in outline the various occasions for the occurrence of that form of self-consciousness which is consciousness of the dominant and triumphant self. In all the cases mentioned, such a consciousness is called out in relation to some sort of opposition which is overcome. No doubt these different forms of the sense of power may occur according to circumstances in various orders of sequence in the developing human life. In racial history the earliest form of it was, as we have tried to show, in physical combat with other members of the same species. But in the course of the development of the individual human life as we know it actual physical combat does not occur as an important factor. The relations of adjustment and opposition to other selves, which evoke self-consciousness, are of a more subtle character. In the human being, who has as the result of racial history inherited imaginative and intellectual capacity in a certain degree, it is possible for these more subtle relations to evoke self-consciousness and pride. We shall complete our account of the will to power from the point of view of feeling more satisfactorily, if we endeavour very briefly to sketch the course of such development.

We start in the first place with the fact that the infant has needs and impulses of its own, chiefly organic cravings for food, warmth, and light. For the satisfaction of these needs it is dependent to a very large extent on adjustment to the movements of external objects. It can carry out movements of its own which either directly cause, or indirectly carry with them, change of visual and other sensations in desired directions, while on the other hand many changes of sensation occur as imposed by external movement, on which the movements of its own body have had no influence. Thus very early there must arise the awareness of a relation between its own impulses and needs with the bodily movements which express them, and on the other hand the resistance or assistance to them given by external force. In this process of learning a differentiation must soon be made between two sorts of external objects. In the first place there is the inanimate thing, which is either unmoving, or else so regular in its movements that only stereotyped sorts of reactions and adjustments are needed to deal with it. On the other hand there are living, and especially human, beings which are distinguishable in a number of ways. The living person appears in many ways to adapt itself spontaneously to further the wishes of the child, without having to be moved by direct manipulations as things have to be. Grown-up persons are perpetually intervening to satisfy requirements which the child cannot fulfil at all or can only fulfil in part by its own unaided activity. Their action thus fits into its own as its continuation and completion.[1] In all forms of co-operative work, as must be obvious, movements and efforts have to be adjusted to the similar but slightly different movements of others. To take part in any sort of co-operation must tend to carry with it the sense of a self co-existing with and in relation to other selves, and it is natural that the unresponsive inanimate thing should be separated off as belonging to a different order. Other human beings also control in many ways the course of the child's experience, e.g. by carrying it about ; and they can deny the fulfilment of its wishes. Thus they appear as sources of dominating power as well as of co-operative help. Moreover persons are capricious and uncertain as compared with things. Regular customs of treatment can be adopted in regard to things with a certainty of the same result always following, whereas the experiences and gestures of other persons have to be carefully watched, and much more subtle and varied forms of adjustment to them have to be adopted. According to circumstances, the same person may either co-operate with or thwart the wishes of the child. Thus persons become much more exciting and interesting objects of attention than things, and a certain capriciousness and spontaneity come to be regarded as their attributes as compared with things. To the above we must add that these beings, which appear as sources both of assistance

[1] See Stout, *Groundwork of Psychology*, 171, who develops this point.

and of impediment and, as apparently capricious and spontaneous, are both exciting and interesting, also show movements which in their form are closely similar to the child's own and can be immediately cognized as such. In these various ways there grows up in the child's mind an idea of himself as a self in relation to a world of other selves and of both as distinguished from the inanimate. Perhaps the most important of the relations in which the self stands to other selves is that which moves between subjection and dominance and gives rise to the varying feelings of depression or humility and elation. Those situations of subjection, in which the child finds himself so often, begin, as his self-consciousness grows, to evoke a reaction of self-assertion. At a stage in childish growth we have the phenomena of contrary suggestion or mere wilfulness, when it is enough for something to be suggested by an elder for the child to refuse or do the opposite.[1] Later on there comes a time when children consciously set before themselves the ideal of being grown up and " able to do what they like ". It has been asserted by Baldwin that this impulse to self-assertion springs from imitation of others. The child observes, so he says, the apparent capriciousness of the behaviour of others (as stated above) and tries to recreate in himself the same phenomenon, endeavouring to be a source of action other than what is expected, and striving after the position of being able to do what he likes.[2] It can certainly be agreed that the child does imitate other persons in this and in other ways and that thus he expands and enriches his own sense of selfhood and agency. But it is surely impossible to believe that self-assertive pride is created *e nihilo* in this manner. Our argument in the foregoing has been directed to prove that it springs from the fundamental elements of mind. Simultaneously,

---

[1] Stern thinks there are signs of this even in the first year, *Psychology of Early Childhood*, 477.

[2] Baldwin, *Mental Development* (1915), 318–24. Still less could we admit that self-consciousness owes its origin to imitation : see Baldwin, loc. cit., and *Social and Ethical Interpretations*, 532.

the experience of selfhood and causative agency is also occurring in the relations of the child to inanimate objects, on which he impresses his will, and in the achievement of mastery over the bodily movements. But always the way in which the experiences both of self-assertive pride and of subjection occur most notably is in the relations to other people. As the child grows, he begins to divide the persons with whom he has to deal into two classes, those to whom he must submit, and those who he can dominate or control. The former attitude is adopted towards parents and elders generally, frequently however with a certain protest, shown in such conduct as deliberate wilfulness and disobedience. The latter tends to be adopted towards other children, particularly those younger than himself. There is, so it is generally held, a period from about the sixth to the tenth year when the attitude of admiration and deference towards elders predominates ; it is the " hero-worshipping " period. From about the tenth year there is a growing tendency to self-assertion and to criticism of elders and teachers. But at all times there are present both the tendencies named. As the child grows and comes into contact with constantly widening circles, he carries on into them the same tendency to measure himself with others and to regard them either with deference or with superiority. McDougall has admirably described this process and its changes of outlook in the growing person who passes from the family to the school, to the university and to the wider world beyond.[1] His idea of himself is very largely that of a person occupying a certain rank or status in a society, an idea not of course continuously present consciously, but as a subconscious background providing an additional motive or a regulating factor in much of the behaviour of life. There is always one power which specially awakens a sentiment of submissiveness, and that is society as a whole, which, as McDougall expresses it, " looms up vaguely and largely behind all individuals ". " The

[1] McDougall, *Introduction to Social Psychology*, 194 and 195.

child comes gradually to understand his position as a member of society indefinitely larger and more powerful than any circle of his acquaintances, a society which with collective voice and irresistible power distributes rewards and punishments, praise and blame, and formulates its approval and disapproval in universally accepted maxims."[1] Our feelings in regard to a crowd spring from the same source. A large crowd of our fellow-citizens seems to embody our society in a concrete form. It is felt to be something unknown and unaccountable, including many individuals whose character and impulses we have not grasped or fathomed, and which is much stronger than ourselves. Hence the nervousness which from the first almost all men feel when singled out to face the attention of a crowd and called on to try and direct or dominate it in any way, especially by addressing it in speech. Yet here too there is a balance struck between submissiveness and self-assertion. Men naturally rebel against too great a subservience to society. In the desire of fame there is included the effort to make one's own impression on society. And having overcome their original timidity before an audience, men attain to one of the intensest of human pleasures when they dominate and sway a great assembly by the power of speech.

In the result the growing person comes normally to regard himself as a self occupying a position in a society of other selves, which is defined as one of dominance in some directions and of submission in others. This more or less conscious sentiment of the self is one to which the original impulse of self-assertion has contributed the most fundamental and primitive elements, but which has also been modified by having grown up in part through relations of co-operation with other selves, and also by the influence of those sympathetic and altruistic impulses which we shall deal with later.

It would seem however that in regard to the foregoing there is need to define somewhat more closely the relations

[1] McDougall, op. cit., 196.

between the impulses of self-assertion and submission. We find that some psychologists speak of self-assertion and self-abasement as " twin instincts which with their affects of positive and negative self-feeling (elation and depression) are normally excited by the cognitions of relative superiority and inferiority to another person ".[1] Is this mode of speaking justified ? I find it difficult to see how it can be supposed that there are two instincts, one to self-assertion and one to self-abasement, which are co-equal, standing on the same level. In general it must be affirmed that the tendency of self-assertion must be prior to any submissive tendency. From the beginning every living thing has only existed by asserting itself and refusing to give way to others ; and the tendency that develops from this is one to aim at the situation of cognized superiority accompanied by its affect of elation. The situation of inferiority to another, on the other hand, is one that is imposed by the superior force of that other ; it is not one that is sought. As soon as we recognize superior force and give way, there is no further impulse to be satisfied. It is always possible to yield in a combat ; and the yielding can hardly be called a separate instinct. The act of submission is moreover accompanied by feeling with an unpleasant tone, which can only be due to the fact that an impulse, that of self-assertion, has been thwarted in its aim, whereas successful self-assertion is accompanied by pleasure, because an instinctive impulse has worked itself out to its due end. Submission and the depression-feeling which goes with it are of course often accompanied by fear, but must be distinguished from it. The course of the fear impulse is this : there occurs an initial depression of vitality, or a set-back to the working out of some instinctive conation, with a prevision of some-thing worse to follow ; and this is followed by the effort to avoid or escape from what appears as the cause of the set-back, and thus to restore the normal course of life. It is therefore in essence an impulse of self-maintenance.

[1] Tansley, *New Psychology*, 188; cf. Drever, *Instinct in Man*, 191.

L

Submission is nothing but the negative of self-assertion ; it is the giving up of self-assertion, accompanied by the opposite feeling, that of pride negated or taken down. It does not seem right therefore to call it an original and positive instinct of human nature, though of course in experience the attitude of submission may become habitual before a power which has often proved itself superior to the agent. It may be said that submission does appear sometimes to be pleasant, for instance, when we submit and reconcile ourselves to our society after a period of opposition and estrangement. The fact can however be easily explained by two considerations. In the first place there is undoubtedly a pleasure sometimes found in relaxing from the strain of self-assertion, in the giving up of pretensions. This tendency does exist in life, but I think we can say of it that it is one which is in contradiction to the essential impulse of life. In so far as, because of opposition and the strain of struggling against it, we yield and give up the struggle, we are acquiescing in a lower level of conscious life. The reason why one who thus gives up the struggle can make his life quite pleasant is as a rule because he finds some other forms of occupation in which various innate tendencies of his nature find easy outlet and satisfaction, not involving the tension of serious conflict. The actual renunciation or yielding itself is a momentary act, an act of acquiescence rather than of active seeking, and the pleasure which it yields can only be a momentary one, being due to the fact of escape from a state of unpleasant fatigue or strain. In the second place submission is pleasant, when it includes the merging of the self in some degree with the stronger and overcoming power, and thus involves the satisfaction of the gregarious instinct. This instinct we shall be dealing with later. Here it may be sufficient to describe it as the impulse to unite oneself as a member with a larger body of one's own species, i.e. a herd or society, and to admit its ends, and a dissatisfaction and unrest when one is felt to be isolated, either physically or mentally, from that body. As a matter of fact, mere submission, in itself a purely negative attitude, always, it would seem, issues into some further positive impulse, either that of fear, to escape from the stronger adversary, or that to adopt in some form the ends of the superior power. If an animal, one of the canine tribe, for example, is worsted in fighting for a piece of food with an animal of another species, his state of mind is rather a compound of anger and fear than a state of submission. The attitude is quite different in face of the leader of his own pack. He flees from the stronger adversary of another species. He still adheres to the company of his stronger leader. A child submits to his parents and does so with some pleasure in the sense of dependence, because he thinks of himself as one of the same circle with them. When we submit to the judgment of our society, we identify ourselves with it and make its ends into our ends.

It might be alleged that a possible case in which submission by itself is experienced as pleasant is that in which a man, worsted in a contest, either serious or playful, is prepared to admit in a generous and " sporting " spirit the superior merit of his adversary. In as far however as there is any admiration of the performance of another, there is always, I think, present an element of " self-projection ", by which we appropriate his performance sympathetically to ourselves. It is perhaps worth while to look briefly at this matter of admiration, for though it takes us away from the gregarious instinct, it is closely related to our general discussion of self-feeling. Admiration has been described by McDougall as wonder combined with negative self-feeling.[1] It includes, that is to say, the appearance of something other than expected, inducing an impulse to explore further and understand more fully, and also the apprehension of some manifestation of qualities, such as strength or skill, beyond our own capacity, which therefore abases our self-feeling. In some cases of admiration, when the phenomenon or the per-

[1] *Introduction to Social Psychology*, 129.

formance is something which we cannot expect to imitate, it is perhaps possible that such a pure self-abasement may be found. But in almost every case it does seem to me that there is some sympathetic appropriation of the admired phenomenon, that is to say a sympathetic echo of the emotions, whether of power or of some other sort, which we read as existing in our object. If it were not so, the contemplation of the admired person or thing would hardly be pleasing. Even in watching the speed of the greyhound or the flight of the eagle, what gives us pleasure is the sympathetic echo of power. In these cases we have something closely related to the sublime. The accepted view of the feeling of sublimity is that it includes two " moments " or phases, first a feeling of abasement or oppression before what is great or powerful, then a reaction in which we take part in, or appropriate to ourselves sympathetically, the power perceived, and so our own self-feeling is raised to a higher intensity.[1] The two phases can hardly be said to be divided temporally, so that we can say that at one point of time there is depression, and at another time elation. It is rather the case that the two tendencies are in a continuous state of interaction. Nevertheless we are, I think, entitled to suggest that the pleasurableness of the sublime is linked with the " moment " of elation, rather than with that of depression. This would certainly be the general opinion in writings on the subject.[2] In the feeling of the sublime the depression tendency appears as subordinate, and only essential because it issues in, and is constantly overcome by, the moment of elation. What is the predominant factor in the total feeling is a sense of being " lifted up ", of sharing in the experience of something greater than oneself. One's own sense of littleness remains, but it is in a state of being constantly transcended. It is the elation phase that tends throughout to be the final or resulting one.

[1] See, for example, Ribot, *Psychology of the Emotions*, 348–51.
[2] See Ribot, loc. cit.

From this digression we may resume the account of the self-assertive impulse as developed in the individual life. It must be admitted that often active ambition seems to be called into existence by experiences of defeat or humiliation. A child passes from the narrow circle of the family, where he has been of some importance, to the school or the outside world, and both finds himself of less importance and also may sustain defeat when he measures himself in some sort of rivalry with those he meets. The bitterness of the blow to his self-esteem may be often a surprise even to himself. A stronger desire for pre-eminence is thus aroused than would have been the case without the defeat. If success comes, the pleasure of it seems proportionately greater ; and so it may go on as wider circles are entered, any failure seeming to add fuel to the desire of success. There are psychologists, of whom Adler is the best known, who find that the initial consciousness of some weakness or deficiency, usually physical, on the part of the child gives the starting-point for the development of all self-assertive tendencies. Thus he states : " One may easily detect in every instance from observation of the child and from the anamneses of the adult that the possession of definitely inferior organs is reflected upon the psyche—and in such a way as to lower the self-esteem, to rouse the child's psychological uncertainty ; but it is just out of this lowered self-esteem that there arises the struggle for self-assertion which assumes forms much more intense than one would expect ".[1] Yet it must be obvious that, for an inferiority to be felt as humiliating and unpleasant, there must have pre-existed some impulse towards self-assertion, even if only in a latent or subconscious form. What may happen in such a case no doubt is this, that in the struggle to escape the lowered self-feeling due to consciousness of inferiority or failure, a greater effort is called out than would have been the case if things had always been felt to go successfully. This effort, once elicited, will tend to

[1] Adler, *The Neurotic Constitution*, (1918), 3.

continue beyond the point at which an initial failure is repaired and equality with others is felt to be restored. It will be carried over by insensible gradations into an aggressive effort towards others, an effort towards "maximation of the ego-consciousness" by means of superiority successfully asserted. But I think it would be generally felt to be somewhat extravagant to assert that all ambition must be due to some initial sense of inferiority, some experiences of failure and humiliation undergone early in life. In the early experiences of childhood, as already described, the varying modes of self-feeling are inevitably called out. It being assumed that a tendency to self-assertion is thus already in existence, a mind conscious of exceptional vigour and of capacities superior to others will be very strongly inclined to measure itself against, and compete with, others in any sphere in which it finds itself. Successes, if they occur, together with the accompanying emotion of elation, will supply sufficient stimulus for the continuance and increase of the effort. We must also allow for the influence exercised by reading and hearing about the successes and the fame of other men in the past and in the present. To a vigorous mind, already motived to some extent by self-assertive pride, such fame may take on something of the appearance of a challenge and a limitation of its own importance. It may thus help to call out an effort to surpass it.

It is no doubt difficult to draw the line between the normal and the abnormal in these cases. But one may perhaps be permitted to surmise that the self-assertiveness which springs from a sense of constitutional inferiority usually shows a restless and unbalanced character which borders on the neurotic. It is a sort of vanity, less secure of itself than the ambition of pure strength, and demanding more constant recognition from others. Thus we find Ludwig in his recent biography of Kaiser Wilhelm II attributes the character of the Emperor largely to the effect of consciousness of his withered arm. The following

extracts, which I take from autobiographical notes in the
life of J. A. Symonds (by H. F. Brown), seem a good
example of self-assertiveness due to a sense of inferiority
and taking on a somewhat unbalanced character. " I
was a physically insignificant boy with an ill-sounding
name, and nothing to rely on in the circumstances of my
family. Instead of expanding in the environment around
me, I felt myself at a disadvantage, and early gained the
notion that I must work for my own place in the world,
in fact that I should have no place till I had made one for
myself. . . . The inborn repugnance to sordid things,
which I have already described as one of my marked
characteristics, now expressed itself in a morbid sense
of my physical ugliness, common patronymic, undistinguished status, and mental ineffectiveness. I did not
envy the possessors of beauty, strength, birth, rank, or
genius, but I vowed to raise myself somehow or other to
eminence of some sort." Again, after speaking of ill-
health and inability to play games at school, he says :
" My external self in these many ways was being perpetually snubbed, crushed, and mortified. Yet the inner
self hardened after a dumb and blind fashion. I kept
repeating : ' Wait, wait, I will, I shall, I must.' "[1]
Yet inferences from such scattered indications as can be
found in the biographies of well-known men can hardly
be used to prove any general theory, one way or the
other. It would be practically impossible to make an
investigation on such lines sufficiently exhaustive.

There is, it must be added, another meaning often
given, or implied, to the expression " self-maximation ".
It is used to mean a will for all-round self-culture, for the
development of all the various human capacities in a
harmonious personality. If this exists as a conscious
human motive, it is only at the highest intellectual levels,
even of human beings, nor could it exist, unless the other
instinctive impulses were already present, each with its

[1] *Life of J. A. Symonds*, by H. F. Brown, Vol. I, 63 ff., 74.

driving force. We do not go into this question here, as it concerns an intellectual level on which we have hardly touched. The will to self-maximation in the narrower sense, i.e. to power, is a mental factor which, as we have seen, derives from far down in the animal world.

CHAPTER V

THE instincts we have hitherto dealt with have all had relation to the maintenance of the life of the individual agent. We have now to turn to that important class of actions which show that some interest is felt for the lives of others than the agent. The actions are those comprised under such general terms as those of altruism or sympathy. It is a difficult task in view of the immense literature on the subject and the wide discrepancies between theories. An outline is all that we can attempt.

An altruistic action, regarded from the outside, is one which has for its object, not the maintenance or forwarding of the agent's own life, as is the case with the instincts hitherto described, but the maintenance or forwarding of the life of another living being, sometimes, but not always, at the sacrifice of some instinctive end of the agent's own. The specific emotion by which this is accompanied, forming part of the internal side of the act, is tender emotion, as it is usually called, directed towards the object of assistance. While we have endeavoured to give some analysis of this emotion in treating of the sexual instinct, it will generally be agreed that, like all other primary emotions such as anger or fear, it contains at its core a shade of feeling which is not capable of further analysis or definition, though all can recognize it.

There are to be observed in children from a very early age isolated acts of compassion or assistance, which seem plainly to bear the marks of being spontaneous and instinctive. There is to be noted the " sharing " that is often practised after the first year of age. " The child's desire to let others share in an enjoyment which he has himself is evidently quite elementary. . . . We all know how children like to hand some of their cake or rolls to other people."[1] Children also show fellow-feeling in passing on toys to others to play with, sometimes to adults, who are quite unsuitable. Childish altruism also often takes the form of the wish to be of practical service. As all know, there is nothing which a child loves more than to assist his elders in their household occupations.[2] No doubt in this something must be put down to the influence of self-feeling. To think that he is assisting his elders and playing his part in their work increases the child's feeling of self-importance. But at the same time the wish to serve or benefit others must be also effective. Both impulses work in the same direction. The suffering of others, or that which appears as suffering, is that which calls out the tender emotions of the child in the strongest form. Many stories could be told to illustrate the spontaneous nature of childish compassion. Sympathy is even shown for the non-real, that is to say for living beings depicted in picture or story, the distinction between reality and representation being often not clearly drawn by the child. Miss Shinn states that the first sign of imaginative sympathy shown by the child whom she observed was in the twenty-fifth month, when the child, looking at a picture of a lamb caught in briars, made a movement to lift away the branch from it.[3] It was just at this period, as Miss Shinn records, that the child was herself showing a strong dislike of being caught, held, or impeded, i.e. a strong desire for bodily freedom. The sympathetic feeling was directed towards the object as to one believed to be similar to herself. Even inanimate objects may call out the child's pity. " When dolls are cut out of paper, the child weeps violently in the most pitiful manner for fear that a head may be cut off. This behaviour calls to mind the cries of ' arme Wiebak '

[1] Stern, *Psychology of Early Childhood*, 527.
[2] Sully (*Studies of Childhood*, 246) illustrates this by a story of a boy aged 2 years 2 months.
[3] Shinn, *Notes on the Development of a Child*, I, 188 and 104.

(poor biscuit) when a biscuit is divided, and ' arme Holz ' (poor wood) when a stick of wood is thrown on the stove. No one has taught the child anything of that sort."[1] No doubt there is an obverse to this picture. Children often appear as totally unfeeling towards suffering, sometimes as cruel to animals or younger children, and often as jealous of their equals. It is not perhaps necessary to go into great detail on this matter. Lack of sympathy is of course due to failure to understand the expressive signs of suffering, especially those given by animals, and thus follows from insufficient experience and undeveloped intellectual powers. Positive cruelty, or what appears as such, appears to be mostly due to curiosity and the attraction of exercising power over other living beings, combined with lack of understanding that suffering is being caused. In envy and jealousy we see self-assertive impulses working against those of altruism. This is a form of conflict of impulses which begins very early. The development of the altruistic tendencies which takes place with growth is to a great extent dependent on intellectual advance and accumulation of experience. There is acquired a further knowledge of the causes and signs of suffering in others, and also, inasmuch as the growing person is attaining a deeper self-consciousness and realization of his own character, there comes a fuller appreciation of the separate character and personality of others, which has to be respected. The case is however not entirely one of intellectual advance ; for it would also seem that about the age of puberty there does take place a certain rather abrupt maturation of altruistic impulses together with a deepening of the tender emotions. But of this it will be more convenient to speak as we pass to discuss the sentiments of love.

The instances thus given are of isolated actions of compassion or of assistance to other individuals who appear to be in some need. There also appear in the course of the individual human development fixed tendencies

---

[1] Preyer, *Mind of the Child*, II, 161.

to feel tender emotion towards, and to exercise some care for, particular individuals. A fixed tendency to experience a certain sort of emotional tendency (fear, anger, tender emotion, etc.) towards a particular object has been in recent English psychology usually called a sentiment. But this term is not usually employed unless the tendency has grown up through habit and experience during the individual life. It has not been used where the tendency seems to be based immediately on instinct, as is the case in parental love. It is proposed to use it here to denote a fixed emotional tendency towards an individual object, apart from the fact whether such tendency may be considered to be the result of individual experience or of an inherited instinct.

A division can be made of the types of altruistic sentiment going with the various relations within the family group. There are the feelings of children to parents, between brothers and sisters as equals, between sexual partners (husband and wife), and of parents to children ; that is to say the filial, fraternal, conjugal, and parental types of sentiment, as we may call them. The above is indeed the order in which they appear in the individual life.

The filial relationship is the first in which the human being is placed in regard to other human beings. The helpless infant, just separated from the maternal organism, hardly exists at first as a separate being ; it is completely dependent on maternal or other care. As its consciousness of itself grows, it comes to realize its close dependence on the care of another. This tendency is not of course personal to the mother. It can be felt in regard to any person who cares for the child. There is felt the strongest need of close physical attachment to, or constant companionship with, some protecting adult. Terror and unhappiness are shown at isolation. The sense of weakness and dependence on others is thus the dominant note in the filial relation. But springing, as it would seem, from this need of protection, there soon arises a special concern for those individuals from whom the child receives it. " The objects of the child's affection are those who satisfy his need of protection and help, of tenderness and care."[1] A child is apt to resent a pretended attack or blow on its mother in a special manner, and, where it understands or believes that the mother is suffering, may attempt consolation.

Though the child shows this tendency most strongly at first towards the protecting adult, he also begins to show it towards other human beings, and this introduces us to what we may term the fraternal type of love, i.e. that which involves, not dependence on, but some sort of equality with, others. While the chief object of the child's love and tenderness is his mother, the circle grows wider until it includes the father, brothers and sisters, near relatives, guardian or nursemaid, later even the kindergarten teacher and playfellows. " It may be said in general that people with whom the child is connected by frequent association are all regarded by him with feelings of liking, however much these may vary in strength and tone."[2] The gregarious instinct now begins to play some part in life. The young child up to about the beginning of the third year prefers to be with protecting elders and shows no desire for companionship with those of his own age.[3] Thereafter he desires with increasing force to have companions with whom to play and share experiences on a footing of something like equality. He becomes very definitely a " herd animal ". School life, especially where there are organized games, meets this need to a great extent in our societies. Where there is no organized school life, there is a spontaneous tendency, as is well known, especially among growing boys, which leads to the formation of various semi-social organizations, clubs, gangs, etc., which often in the big towns take on a predatory or semi-criminal character. The tendency is seen also in the formation of the student organizations

[1] Stern, op. cit., 508.   [2] Stern, op. cit., 508.
[3] Groos, *Spiele der Menschen*, 432–4.

so common in the universities of many countries.[1]   The
view generally held at present is that there is in man, as
in some other animals, a gregarious instinct, which in itself
is nothing but a craving for the proximity of fellow-beings
of the same species and a discomfort in separation from
them, and does not necessarily include any impulse to
assist such companions when in any distress, the altruistic
impulse being derived from a different instinctive source.
This is a question into which we shall go later.   It is
however plain as a matter of fact that for those who we
reckon as belonging to the same group, and with whom we
are accustomed to co-operate, there is as a rule felt a
special concern.   Their fortunes affect us more intimately
than those of others, and there is a special tendency to
share with them, rather than with others, any good things
which may come in our way.   We may in general describe
the spirit of fraternal love under the term " comradeship ".
It is shown especially in acts of co-operation, mutual
service, and sharing as between equals.

We may see in personal friendship a specialization of
the fraternal type of love to a particular individual in
the form of a fixed sentiment of affection.   One of the
most potent causes of friendship consists in the fact of
the sharing of experiences, particularly if the experiences
are of an especially exciting and interesting character,
such as common danger.   A common work and common
interests are also effective grounds of friendship.   As the
result of some such causes as these, the friends may feel
themselves united in a special bond of unity, and constituting, as it were, a small group or " herd " by itself, distinct
from other similar groups.   A " Triumvirate ", or perhaps
even a larger group, is a possibility, though a special
friendship is as a rule between two only.   As the result
each friend feels a special concern for the interest of the
other, and at the same time realizes more vividly than
with other persons the individual character and person-

---

[1] Many particulars of such groups and organizations are given by
Stanley Hall, *Adolescence*, II, 396–417.

ality of his friend. It becomes something valuable to him, which he will make special efforts to guard against hurt or diminution, efforts which may involve incidentally some sacrifice of valuable ends personal to the agent himself.

At the time of puberty, as we have already remarked, there is a certain deepening of the emotional life, and especially the tendency of the self to go outwards in tender emotion is increased. Stanley Hall has stated that at adolescence there is a striking advance or outgrowth of the mental life in various directions, and amongst them both in the self-assertive and the altruistic tendencies. Self-confidence is increased, the individual becomes more conscious of himself, and as a correlative to this he becomes more vividly aware of the personality of others. At the same time altruistic emotions are intensified. " Self-subordination may become a passion. Youth devotes himself, perhaps by a vow, to a lifetime of self-denial or painful servitude to some great cause or a career in which some of the deepest of human instincts must be mortified and eradicated."[1] " Few sentiments undergo a greater increase of both depth and range at this age than those of sympathy and pity."[2] In these manifestations we may doubtless see what is in the nature of a preparation of the characters which find their full sphere in the conjugal relation and in parenthood. To some extent there is in these relations an interruption and superseding of the pure gregarious instinct, that which seeks association with a body of equal comrades. The relation to the partner and offspring takes its place. We have already made some remarks on sexual love when dealing with the sexual instincts. There is involved in it both a vivid apprehension of the personality of the beloved and a going out of the self in protective tenderness. In the actual conjugal relationship these characters may be further enhanced. In marriage there is, or should be,

---

[1] Stanley Hall, *Adolescence*, II, 81.
[2] Ibid., II, 373.

a strong element of comradeship. All shared experiences and co-operation in any work lead naturally to the formation of a felt bond of union. In the conjugal relation the experiences shared are among the most vivid and interesting in human life. Moreover the functions of the sexes are different both in the procreation and the rearing of offspring ; and in many respects the characters of the sexes are different from and complementary to one another. Hence there must tend to arise on the part of each partner a peculiarly vivid realization of the conscious life of the other as in relation to his or her own. And, inasmuch as the pleasurable activity of the one partner appears as bound up with the conscious life of the other, that conscious life will appear as something valuable, to be protected with special devotion and tenderness.

The starting point of parental love would appear to be, on the part of the mother, a vivid sense of a unity binding the new life in one whole with her own. On the part of the father, this may be felt, though less vividly, as we have already endeavoured to show. It is in the relation of the mother to her child that the element of protective tenderness, present in all love, reaches its highest degree. It has been said that to the mother the infant is a part of herself, and that it is as such that she guards it.[1] But the specific note of tender emotion is not present in regard to what we think of as entirely a part of ourselves. The love of the mother is toward something which, though derived from herself, is regarded as a new and separate life, and it is felt on the part of one who has already been conscious of her own individuality. Tender emotion is indeed that which is felt when an individual, conscious of himself as such, goes out to guard the life of another individual. A mother usually resents her baby being called " it ", and demands the use of " he " or " she ". From the first there is normally a pleasure felt in the sense of the separate conscious life of the child, and this to an increasing extent afterwards. So that we may say there is no

[1] Aristotle, *Ethics*, VIII, 12. 2.

necessary fusing of the bounds of individuality, but rather the reckoning of the two lives as bound together in one whole, in which one plays the part of protector and the other of protected. In the felt contrast with the helpless and appealing life of the child the parent's own sense of personality will be heightened rather than lowered.

The main difference between the maternal and other forms of love would appear to be this, that in the former the protecting activity is more constantly called for and exercised owing to the helplessness of the human infant. In any form of love there may be adopted a watchful and protecting attitude, a readiness to shield the object of love from possible harm, as it is expressed in the poem of Heine, which we quoted above. But this mental attitude will hardly be an element constantly in the foreground of consciousness in other forms of love, as it is likely to be in the maternal tenderness.

The parental instinct of protection is strongest on the part of parents towards their own children, i.e. when it arises as part of the conative train of the reproductive instinct. It is however also felt, though to a lesser degree, towards other infants or towards the helpless young of some other species. There are many strange adoptions recorded on the part of female animals ; sometimes they have adopted and cared for the young of species which are their usual prey, or to which as adults they are bitterly hostile. These facts however hardly justify Herbert Spencer in holding that parental love is only a particular form of a general instinct of tenderness liable to be excited by any living being which is comparatively small and helpless.[1] The better account would seem to be that of McDougall, namely that what takes place is an extension of the parental instinct to something resembling its native object.[2] I do not know if any investigation has been made as to how far down in the animal

---

[1] H. Spencer, *Principles of Psychology*, II, 689–92.
[2] McDougall, *Introduction to Social Psychology*, 73–4.

world the facts of adoption are found. But we are probably justified in believing that, the lesser the degree of intelligence and adaptability in the animal, the more closely is the parental impulse of protection confined to the animal's own offspring, as part of the conative train of reproduction. When we come to animals higher in the scale of intelligence, we find that a strong instinct often acquires a certain independence and, provided it is not satisfied in the normal way, discharges itself on any thing sufficiently resembling its original object. This is the case with the hunting instinct, i.e. the impulse to pursue and capture prey, which is normally a subsidiary part of the instinctive maintenance of the bodily functions through nutrition. Hence when an adult has no children which would satisfy the reproductive instinct, we find there is often the strong impulse to take charge of something small and helpless, the young either of its own species or of one sufficiently like it. Both Herbert Spencer and McDougall remark on how in the human race a sort of tender impulse can even be evoked by anything small and delicate of its kind ; e.g. a woman will speak of a " dear little cup " or " chair," etc.

It will be convenient to say something here of what the Freudian school has called the " ambivalence " of love and hate. By this it is meant that love and hate have a tendency to pass the one into the other, and can be directed simultaneously towards the same object, there being as a rule some repression of the hate tendency. Freud states that " the evidence of psycho-analysis shows that almost every intimate emotional relation between two persons which lasts for some time—marriage, friendship, the relations between parents and children—leaves a sediment of feelings of aversion and hostility, which have first to be eliminated by repression ".[1] The amount of truth in this view would seem to be as follows. Our egoistic tendencies, we feel, are liable to be constantly impeded by the presence of others ; we feel compelled to

[1] Freud, *Group Psychology and the Analysis of the Ego*, 54.

pay attention to them and cannot do exactly as we should otherwise please. " As soon as anyone is near me," Dostoievsky makes one of his characters say, " his personality disturbs my self-complacency and restricts my freedom ".[1] James has labelled this as " the instinct of personal isolation ".[2] But it does not seem necessary to appeal to any separate instinct. There is surely in it nothing more than a form of the egoistic self-maintaining and self-assertive impulse, which finds its expression in other instincts. Our self-assertion may be limited and opposed both by fear of others and also by the instinct which impels us to pay attention to them and feel concern for their interests. Those with whom a person is most closely associated in family life are likely to be just those who are most felt as limiting his power to pursue other ends. It is not very likely that this will be felt by a mother towards her child, as the impulses of tender emotion seem in this case as a rule to be predominant ; but it does happen that a mother sometimes feels her child as a burden and impediment to the pursuit of other instinctive ends which are considered as valuable. In all such cases of a conflict between the self-regarding and other-regarding impulses, even if the impulse of love is predominant on the whole, yet there may still exist, as the psychoanalysts have pointed out, a repressed and half-conscious resentment at the limiting effect of the tie of affection.

There are forms of the sentiment of love with wider or more generalized objects than those mentioned. We will in the first place consider the devotion to, and will to serve, that group of which a man reckons himself a part, patriotism as it is usually called, whether for the nation, or for any smaller group within it, such as town, school, club, etc. This sentiment, as we know it in man, includes two factors. In the first place, as has been already remarked, when one reckons oneself as a member of a

---

[1] *The Brothers Karamazov*, chap. IV.
[2] *Principles of Psychology*, II, 437 and 438.

group, there is as a rule a disposition to feel a special concern for the interests of the individual members of that group as compared with outsiders. An Englishman feels drawn towards another Englishman if he meets him when travelling abroad. A man has a special fellow-feeling for those of his own trade, those who have been at his old school and so on. Such a sentiment depends on the formation of a concept of a certain class including a number of individuals and the power to recognize such individuals by some sign and distinguish them from others. In the second place we find that there takes place in the man who reckons himself a member of a group an extension of the self-sentiment, so that he now identifies himself to a partial extent with a group, held in idea over other similar groups, and concerns himself for its welfare in the same way as for that of his own narrower self. Such an extension may take place with regard to any group of which a man reckons himself a member, his family, town, school, club, etc. But the clearest and perhaps strongest form in which it occurs is in the sentiment for one's country, commonly called patriotism. This extension of the self-regarding sentiment must be distinguished from the pride which a man may take in the objects associated with him on the ground that he has made or contributed to make them. Of this latter sort would be to some extent the pride of a man in his clothes or his house, which he had chosen or designed ; and the pride of parents in their children is partly similar. It is possible to have a sentiment for one's country or other group without any sense of contributing to its actions. An individual onlooker at a football match may feel an intense interest in the victory of his town side, though he has never contributed anything to its formation, or ever played the game. It is not possible, I think, to find any so-called " rational " ground for this impulse. The foundation of it appears to be an innate and irrational urge, which we must think of as connected with the gregarious instinct, to unite oneself as a member with some larger body or " herd " of one's kind. When this union is thought of as effected, and when there is the intellectual capacity to think of this body as a collective whole distinguished from other similar wholes, then it follows that there is a partial identification of the self with it, and the good or ill fortune of this body is treated to some extent as the good or ill fortune of the self. Any qualities which belong in any way to the group and distinguish it from other groups can then be taken as reflecting credit on oneself. It is thus even that merely extraneous qualities, such as the beauty of the scenery of the district or country in which a man lives as compared with the scenery of other localities, can be regarded as appertaining to his group and he comes to have a certain pride in them.[1] Given the operation of this instinctive impulse, the identification of the self with the group is made closer by other factors. The chief cause for such closer identification is to be found in the fact that in some way or other membership of the group makes a practical difference to the life of the member. Even in the case of an isolated tribe of primitive men, having little or no relations with other tribes, it is doubtless the case that any co-operative work, the united effort against the forces of nature or against wild animals, must tend to make men think of the group as a collective whole, with which they identify themselves. This will be still more the case when the group or tribe has relations of any sort with other groups, and the individual finds that, by reason of his membership of a given group, he is treated differently by the members of other groups, that is to say, for the most part with less friendliness and sympathy than by his own fellow-countrymen. Thus ultimately the full-blown spirit

---

[1] One might surmise, I think, that it is due to this instinctive urge that whenever we see two groups or sides engaged in any contest, we can hardly help joining ourselves in sympathy to one side or the other and taking its fortune to heart as our own. Few boys probably can read the *Iliad* without taking a side, usually with the Trojans and Hector. There must be the same unreasoning ground for the fact that a large part of the youth of London were accustomed to count themselves Oxford or Cambridge at the time of the University Boat Race, while having no connection with either University.

of group patriotism comes to be formed, in which a man partially identifies himself with a nation or state, which he thinks of as standing over against a number of other similar nations or states. Speaking generally, the form of the self-feeling in which a man regards himself as forming one with his nation will be that of self-assertive pride, or the will to power. This follows naturally because it is almost entirely through relations of opposition to other forces (whether of nature or of other groups) that awareness of the group as a separate unit is created, and moreover the difference which membership of a given group makes to the individual consists mainly in this, that by co-operative effort some advantage is secured to him in the struggle for existence against the forces of nature, wild animals, or other groups of men. Hence the form which patriotic sentiment naturally takes is that of a will to increase the power, prestige, and glory of one's own nation as against other nations, conceived as rivals or opponents. This is illustrated by the facts of patriotic sentiment as we know them. British Imperialists come for the most part from the outposts of Empire, where they are in constant contact with outsiders, whose conduct towards them is modified by the fact of their citizenship of the Empire. The strongest home of German national feeling has always been Prussia, which came into existence as an outpost of Germanism against the Slavonic tribes, and whose history has been largely determined by the relations based on that fact. But we will consider the nature of the patriotic sentiment further later after first looking at the other and wider forms of altruism.

The other and wider forms of altruistic sentiment find their object in some class of persons, and thus depend on the formation of a concept. Thus we may find a person devote himself to the service of some general class, for example, slaves, crippled children, or those suffering from some particular disease, which excites his sympathy. In the most general forms of all there may be a sentiment for humanity, for man as man, and even for all living beings. In the formation of the concept the class is distinguished intellectually from other classes, but it is not necessary that it should be regarded as a unitary group having actual relations with other groups. In all these cases the general sentiment is dependent on the fact that some concern has first been felt for individuals. For example, a person first feels compassion for some individual crippled child, and then forming an idea of the general class, may determine to devote him or her self to the service of crippled children generally in some hospital or elsewhere. The sentiment for humanity is a generalization depending on the fact that sympathy and the wish to help have first been felt towards individual men. When the general sentiment has been formed, there may perhaps be some danger that the individual may be treated as a mere type, and that the warmth of the sympathetic feeling may be thereby lessened. But this is by no means necessary. To realize that the individual assisted is one of a class may rather carry with it something of an added appeal ; the feeling in taking on a wider character may also be in some degree deepened and intensified. To realize in some degree the tie of our common humanity with the individual need involve no lessening of the intensity of our personal sympathy.

What, it may then be asked, is the relation of these more universal sentiments to the narrower ones, those for the family or for some particular group, and if it be assumed that an extension of altruistic sentiment from the narrower to the more comprehensive forms has taken place, how can we think of such a progress as having been made ? As I conceive the matter, to consider this question of the extension of the altruistic sentiments will help us to analyse further the altruistic impulse itself and arrive at its essential nature, for no theory can be adequate which is not based on the whole of the facts regarding the instinct, its latest as well as its most primitive forms. We therefore propose to consider this question in some detail.

It is possible to think of the patriotic sentiment as

capable of being extended and universalized in respect of each of the two factors of which, as we have pointed out, it is composed. In as far as the group sentiment means that we recognize a bond of union with certain persons, members of our society, it is possible to think of that feeling of union as being extended to a wider sphere, so as to include other individuals outside the group, and in the last resort all members of the human race or all living beings. In this a man's first and most obvious duty may, of course, still remain that to those immediately near him. The primary service of each may still be rendered to his own family and his own immediate circle. Whether patriotic sentiment, regarded as consisting in an extension of the self-sentiment, is capable of being transformed so as to become a universalized sentiment of altruism depends on the form in which it appears. If a man in serving his country is making it his sole end to increase its power as against other groups, that is to say, if the impulse with which he endows that extended self, his country, is solely that of personal pride or self-assertion, it is plain that there is no way by which this form of patriotism can be extended to become a sentiment for humanity.[1] Humanity must appear to such a mind as only composed of warring or rival groups, without a common bond, with one of which he identifies himself. As we have already remarked, it is this form which

---

[1] There was among pre-war German writers a strong tendency to take this point of view. Treitschke wrote as follows : " If we apply the standards of a deeper Christian morality to the State, and if we bear in mind that the essence of this great collective individuality is power, we realize that the highest moral duty of a State is to maintain its power. The individual must be sacrificed for the sake of a higher community of which he is a member. But the State is the supreme human community ; therefore in the case of the State there can be no duty of self-sacrifice." (*The Political Thought of Heinrich von Treitschke*, by H. W. C. Davis, 166–7.) Yet even he seems hardly consistent, for he also writes as follows : " The State is a moral community ; it is called upon to make positive efforts for the education of the human race, and its final aim is that a people may shape for themselves a real character in it and by means of it." (Op. cit., 135.) And again : " The rays of divine light reveal themselves in a broken form in many peoples, each of which manifests a new shape and a new conception of the Godhead." (Op. cit., 129–30.)

patriotic sentiment does tend primarily to take. But it is possible to think of one's country's place in the world in another way, that is to say on the analogy of a self which forms part of a community with other selves and co-operates with them towards common ends. There is always the possibility of thinking of the relations in this way, inasmuch as in the individual in existing society the consciousness of self grows up under the influence not only of relations of opposition to other selves, but also those of co-operation and mutual help. Individaul thinkers in the past have often put forward this idea of a society of nations, and as we know, an endeavour is now being made to realize it in the League of Nations. It means that we conceive of our nation as a member of common end, which may at times be regarded as merely a society co-operating with other nations towards a negative, i.e. the restraint of those self-assertive impulses which would involve the possibility of war, but also may take a positive form, ultimately the raising of the general level of conscious life and happiness throughout the nations of the world.

But to show that it is logically possible for the narrower forms of altruistic sentiment to be extended into wider ones is not the same thing as to give an account of how the extension has actually taken place. It will, I hope, help us to form our general conclusions if we now consider this point.

In much of recent psychology the practice has been to regard all the altruistic impulses as derived from the parental instinct with its tendency of protective tenderness towards the young. The account of the extension of this instinct to other objects, which could be given from an evolutionary point of view, would, I believe, be somewhat on the following lines.[1] In the first place there is the deep-seated parental instinct leading to the care of the

---

[1] This account is mainly derived from H. Spencer, *Principles of Psychology* and *Principles of Sociology*. But it is supplemented by materials suggested by other writers, Westermarck, Sutherland, McDougall.

life of offspring. As already pointed out, amongst many of the higher animals, as well as men, the impulse of this instinct directs itself towards any object sufficiently resembling the helpless young of the same species as the adult, as shown in adoption. With man there begins to be even a further extension, so that tender feeling may be in some cases felt towards another adult, who is helpless or in any distress. The most primitive races live as a rule in widely scattered tribes. They are organized for hunting or to win a livelihood from nature. But these groups do not enter into organized competition with each other. Such quarrels and fights as arise are personal, and organized warfare does not exist. At a later stage, chiefly as the result of closer contact and competition for food supply, wars arise between tribes. In these wars one of the chief factors leading to the victory of one tribe over another was that of internal cohesion or organization. Those tribes in which the individuals were most ready to subordinate their private welfare to that of the group, and most ready to assist any of their fellow-countrymen in need, were likely to prevail and destroy other tribes. Thus there was a selection by inter-tribal warfare (as well as to some extent through the contest with nature) of those tribes in which loyalty to the group and altruistic impulses towards its members were strongest. This process of selection admittedly did not produce a wholly sympathetic and altruistic character, as we conceive it. The inter-tribal struggle produced, as the obverse of devotion to one's own group and its members, fixed tendencies of hostility, fear, or suspicion towards outsiders. To quote one striking fact, in both Greek and Latin the words for enemy, ἐχθρός and hostis, are derived from words meaning nothing more than outsider or stranger ; the words for enemy and for outsider were originally the same. Most savage societies treat strangers quite differently to fellow-citizens. It is often permissible or praiseworthy to take the lives of the former, while it is a crime to take that of a member of the tribe. We see much the same in many animal societies. Moreover within the society it was not only altruistic tendencies that were fostered. Men were likely to treat their fellow-citizens with kindness only in so far as the interests of the tribe called for it. The weak, old, ailing, or otherwise useless were not likely to be treated with consideration for their own sake. It has often been the custom in savage tribes to abandon such persons or even to help them out of life. The type of character produced in the successful warrior state was, in its extreme form (to adapt a phrase used somewhere by Nietzsche), one that was ready to sacrifice either itself or its neighbour with equal ruthlessness to its ideal of the service of its community. Here too there are analogies in animal societies, where there is often the tendency to attack and destroy wounded and ailing members. After this type of the successful warrior state had grown up, there was a tendency to pass beyond it, when the inter-tribal struggles led to the subjection of the conquered and not to their destruction. The victors began to see that it might be more to their advantage to keep their conquered enemies as subjects and tributaries than to massacre them and create a desert by their conquests. Thus large empires grew up, of which the Roman Empire is the greatest example. Within a large empire of this kind, those inhabitants, the great majority, who lived in the interior became accustomed to friendly and co-operative relations with their neighbours ; this was their ordinary milieu. Familiarity with warlike conditions, relations with outsiders and enemies, were confined to a small professional army and to a narrow fringe on the frontiers. Moreover even with strangers and on the frontiers relations of trade began to be more common than those of war. Thus the type of feeling towards outsiders caused by constant fighting against them tended to die out, because so seldom evoked. The sentiments of hostility towards outsiders, fostered by the inter-tribal struggle, tended to fall away as that struggle ceased. They were not based on any fundamental human instinct, but were only the temporary result of accidental conditions. Men do not naturally hate one another, it might be said, but only in so far as accident has brought it about that they have to compete for the same objects, such as food, because there is not enough to go round. Similarly within the State, it was not in accordance with any natural instinct to destroy the unfit ; it was only incidentally necessary because of the pressure on the means of subsistence. On the other hand the general impulses of altruistic tenderness towards the weak and helpless still remained, inasmuch as they were founded in a deep-seated instinct, the parental, essential to the race from its earliest beginnings. This instinct had been moreover strengthened in the course of the inter-tribal struggle, in so far as it was directed to those with whom a man was most in contact, his neighbours. There was thus every reason for it, as it were, to come into its own in the general milieu of peace and toleration. As an auxiliary to these tendencies there has taken place a growth in man of imaginative and representative power, which has meant an increase of the capacity to realize when others are distressed. The awareness through sympathy of another's suffering does not of itself carry with it a will to relieve that suffering. But given an existing impulse to be concerned for others, derived from the parental instinct, then men, as their powers of discrimination and representation grow, will be quicker to note the signs of distress in others and realize what they mean ; so that there will be felt a desire to assist others on more numerous occasions, and the range of the objects for the altruistic impulses will be also increased. At the same time of course within organized communities the mere wish for order, peace, and comfort was a motive causing hatred and violence to be blamed, and love to be extolled. All these tendencies were finally summed up and made explicit in great religions of universal love and benevolence, Buddhism and Christianity ; though even now the supremacy of the altruistic impulses is not established ;

they are often more preached as ideals than followed in practice.

To the acceptance of this account we may oppose two considerations which seem to give reason for doubt. The first concerns the question of origin and raises what is perhaps rather a far-reaching question of principle. The theory given has to start with the supposition that the parental instinct was in origin a small accidental variation, and that it is this which has been developed by natural selection. A congenital variation, as it is assumed to occur in the Darwinian theory of evolution, means some small modification of the physical structure ; and it is, I suppose, conceivable that such a modification might carry with it some variation in the pattern or order of the movements of the animal concerned, which might at the same time involve also a slightly modified emotional consciousness. But it does not seem conceivable that a quite new pattern and organization of behaviour should appear in this way, that is to say, an activity devoted to a new sort of end, and accompanied by a new sort of feeling. It must be admitted, unless all life is a mechanism or an automatism, that there is a will or effort on the part of the organism towards the preservation of its individual life, which, as we have expressed it, means the maintenance of a certain series of bodily sensations. This impulse cannot itself be the result of an accidental variation, aided by natural selection ; for the struggle for existence presupposes the individual will to live. It is not conceivable then that the will to maintain and protect another life can be in any sense an accidental variation. It must be either the natural outgrowth and continuation of the individual will to live, or be the result of another parallel principle present in life from its earliest beginning.

Our second objection concerns the nature of the final stage of the process, a stage which has indeed for the most part taken place in historical times and is open to observation. The account given hardly seems adequate to the way in which an extended altruistic morality has been adopted. It would be a somewhat anomalous fact if an instinct, the intensification and extension of which had up to a point been due to the workings of the struggle for existence and natural selection, should, just at the time when those factors ceased to operate, show a somewhat abrupt increase in strength, at least in certain individuals, and come to be adopted as an ideal rule of life with so much enthusiasm (at least in theory) by many following them.[1] We seem to find in fact that a doctrine of humanitarianism, of the value of human life in itself, apart from divisions of nationality and race, has been adopted, in so far as it has been adopted, with a passion of enthusiasm to which, on the account given, we lack a clue. The spirit of which we speak is that shown, for example, in the English movement for the abolition of negro slavery, and which still inspires the attitude of most civilized men towards slavery. It is not necessarily connected with Christian beliefs, for many who reject Christianity, e.g. the Positivists, hold the same ethics with at least equal fervour. If what we are in presence of here was only the gradual development of an instinct (one among many, the result of an accidental variation), and its intensive appearance (also accidental) in certain individuals, it is difficult to see why those individuals, e.g. Buddha or St. Francis, should not in the first place have been received with a shock of mere surprise as freaks or abnormal examples of a certain normal characteristic. It would be difficult to find reasons why the religion of universal love should have carried an immediate and passionate acceptance on the part of so many, seeming as it were to appeal to something which was only waiting to be called out. It would also appear to follow, in default of some further explanation, that the sentiment of love in becoming universalized would always and necessarily also have become weaker. No doubt it is true of many that their most intense devotion is to

[1] See Green, *Prolegomena to Ethics* (1906), 239, where a similar argument is used.

individuals or to a narrow circle, and that to wider circles there is either indifference or a much weaker sort of feeling. But there are also many others who feel the appeal of the widest sentiments of love without any diminution of its intensity. As we have already remarked, the feeling in directing itself towards a wider or more conceptualized object becomes in their case at the same time deepened and strengthened. Work conceived as for the benefit of a whole nation or even for that of mankind is likely then to be carried on with more devotion than that for a narrow circle. Even if benevolent impulses are only able to find practical application towards particular individuals, those individuals need not be regarded with any less warmth of feeling because there is some more or less conscious realization of the tie of a common humanity. What would be often regarded as one of the highest expressions of this spirit is that of Dante : " That infinite and unspeakable Good which dwells on high is attracted to love even as a ray of light to a luminous body. It communicates its ardour in proportion to what it finds ; so that the more widely love extends, the greater is the measure in which God's grace is imparted to it : and according as the number of harmonious spirits above is greater, there are more objects of pure love, and more love is felt there and this is reflected as by a mirror from one to the other."[1] It was of this passage that Shelley was thinking when he wrote the lines in " Epipsychidion " which begin :

> True love in this differs from gold and clay
> That to divide is not to take away.
>
> .   .   .   .   .
>
> This truth is that deep well whence sages draw
> The unenvied light of hope, the eternal law
> By which those live to whom this world of life
> Is as a garden ravaged, and whose strife
> Tills for the promise of a later birth
> The wilderness of this elysian earth.

[1] Dante, " Purgatorio," Canto XV. (Tozer's translation.)

There can be no mistaking the intensity of feeling that lies behind these lines.

Still less on the theoretical account given above is it easy to account for the fact that a sentiment of kinship, not only with all humanity, but with all the world of living animals, has been felt, and a regard for animals accordingly adopted as a principle. Christianity has never, in theory at least, laid much stress on the kinship of men with animals. For the strongest expressions of this sentiment we have to turn to Eastern religions. The Koran has the following : " There is not a beast upon the earth, nor a bird that flieth with both its wings, but is a nation like to you . . . to their Lord shall they be gathered ".[1] Rabindranath Tagore writes as follows (referring to the adoption of Buddhism in India) : " In the west the prevalent feeling is that nature belongs exclusively to inanimate things and to beasts, that there is a sudden unaccountable break where human nature begins. According to it everything that is low in the scale of beings is merely nature, and whatever has the stamp of perfection on it, intellectual or moral, is human nature. . . . But the Indian mind never has any hesitation in acknowledging its kinship with nature, its unbroken relation with all. The fundamental unity of creation was not simply a philosophical speculation for India ; it was her life object to realize this great harmony in feeling and action. . . . This was the reason why in India a whole people, who once were meat-eaters, gave up taking animal food to cultivate the sentiment of universal sympathy for life, an event unique in the history of mankind."[2] It is not easy to see what preparation there could have been for sentiments of this kind during the periods of inter-tribal struggle for existence ; for man only required to tend the animals in so far as they were useful to him, and at no time would compassion for them have been useful for survival.

---

[1] Koran, c. 6.   [2] Tagore, *Sadhana*, 6-9.

Can we then give some account of the origin and essential nature of the altruistic impulses other than that sketched above ? In order to make this attempt we must, I think, first look further at the gregarious instinct. The gregarious instinct is usually described as an impulse which has its goal merely in the near presence of other individuals of the same species and which avoids isolation ; it is described as carrying with it a primary unanalysable sense of comfort in the actual presence of comrades, and a similar sense of discomfort in their absence.[1] This mere love of companionship, it is usually held, does not necessarily involve any impulse towards the protection or assistance of the companions. The quotation is often made of the description of the Damaraland ox by Galton. " Yet although the ox has so little affection for or individual interest in his fellows, he cannot endure even a momentary severance from his herd. If he be separated from it by stratagem or force, he exhibits every sign of mental agony, he strives with all his might to get back again, and when he succeeds, he plunges into its middle to bathe his whole body with the comfort of closest companionship."[2] The perceptual situation which the instinct strives to maintain is thus that which can be described under the terms " proximity to living animals of own species ". The conative impulse of the instinct is disturbed by the disappearance of the companions and the resulting isolation, and thus will cause effort, accompanied by unpleasure, to restore the perceptual situation of companionship. But it seems plain that the instinctive impulse must also suffer some frustration and disturbance if the companions themselves are affected in some way. Companionship is sought with fellows, not dead or ailing, but living and in normal vigour. It must be admitted that the impulse to companionship will be subject to some sort of shock when the companions,

---

[1] See Trotter, *Instincts of the Herd*, 31. McDougall, *Outline of Psychology*, 154.
[2] Galton, *Enquiries into Human Faculty*, 72.

N

or any of them, suffer damage or death ; and some sort
of a conation may be aroused towards restoration of the
normal perceptual situation. When the impulse to herd-
fellowship is disturbed by isolation, the means of restoration are simple ; the herd has only to be looked for again.
In this, the simplest form of the instinct, it appears as
nothing more than a fear of isolation. When however
the instinct is disturbed by some injury to the members of
the herd, restoration of the normal situation calls for more
developed intellectual capacity. In the first place there is
needed the power to realize sympathetically the circumstances of the distressed comrade ; and so among the
less intelligent animals we could only expect to find
concern at the distress of their comrades where the injury
is of some obvious character. And in the second place,
in such cases some insight is usually required into the cause
of the injury before action can be taken in order to deal
with it. It is for these reasons, we may surmise, that it is
only amongst the more intelligent of gregarious animals
that there are to be observed attempts to assist companions when in distress. There are of course great
varieties in the degree of intelligence required according
to circumstances. Hudson records that, when South
American vizcachas are sealed up in their burrows by
human agency, other vizcachas come often from a distance
to dig them out. The vizcachas are, he says, extremely fond
of each other's society, and hence, it may be, the desire to
see, as usual, their buried neighbours becomes intense
enough to impel them to work their way to them.[1] Whatever be the correct explanation, it is plain that the impulse
to companionship and that to assistance of the comrade
work in the same direction, and in any case no high degree
of insight into the cause of the distress is required. We may
say the same perhaps for any attempts to set free im-
prisoned comrades, as, for instance, of the cases related
by Livingstone in which elephants combined to lift young

---

[1] Hudson, *Naturalist in La Plata*, 311 and 312.

comrades out of the pits in which they had been
entrapped.[1] There is however a great body of evidence
to show that gregarious animals do in more complex
cases show concern for the well-being of their fellows and
assist them in ways which show some insight into the
cause of injury or threatened injury; and it is certain
that non-gregarious animals do not do this in the same way,
except for their young or mates. " It is certain ", writes
Darwin, " that associated animals have a feeling of love
for one another which is not felt by non-social adult
animals."[2] Darwin and others give a large number of
instances in support of this assertion.[3] Many gregarious
species, especially of the sheep and goat tribes, warn
each other of danger; many herbivorous animals defend
each other from attack, and instances are recorded
in which assistance is given to comrades, when
wounded, and animals, who have been disabled and are
unable to feed themselves, have been supplied with
food by their companions. A striking instance of this
last sort given by Darwin is that an old and completely
blind pelican was found on a salt lake in Utah; it was
very fat and must have been well fed for a long time by
its companions. Man in domesticating the dog has availed
himself of the same instinct. It is plain that the dog
adopts the members of his household as his " herd ",
and we need not say how he often resents injury to them
and will defend them from attack. Monkeys do the same;
when in captivity they have been known to defend a
keeper, to whom they are attached, from the attack of
another monkey.[4] No doubt a distinction is to be drawn
between the mere satisfaction in the proximity of others
and the active concern for individual members of the
group. The former supplies a constant background to
the life of the gregarious animal and is a continuous and
permanent motive from which springs under exceptional

[1] Quoted by Sutherland, *Origin and Growth of Moral Instinct*, I, 327.
[2] Darwin, *Descent of Man*, 155.
[3] Darwin, op. cit., 153–9; and see Sutherland, op. cit., I, 300–48.
[4] See e.g. Darwin, op. cit., 157–8.

circumstances the will to help distressed members of the group. Köhler records of the chimpanzees observed by him that, when one is separated and put in a cage by himself, he shows intense mental distress and endeavours to get back to his comrades. The others are not so miserable over the separation as he is ; they are still the " group ", but do show *some* signs of concern and sympathy. When the separated animal is returned to the main body, he shows intense excitement and pleasure, the others, though less excited, do show signs of satisfaction.[1] It seems plain that the main interest of the gregarious animal is usually in the group of his associates as a whole and not in any particular individual. But the group is composed of individuals and, if they were removed singly, no group would be left. Any diminution of the group by separation of or injury to an individual does in fact seem *pro tanto* to have some disturbing effect on the gregarious instinct.

A fact that has to be allowed for is that some gregarious animals, cattle and dogs especially, show not infrequently an impulse to attack and destroy, not to assist, wounded members of their herd. This impulse has been a good deal discussed, but its exact significance seems somewhat doubtful. Hudson was of opinion that the perception of an injured comrade arouses a defensive impulse in the form of a furious wish to attack something ; if there is no other agent to be observed at the time, the members of the herd may in their blind fury attack their injured comrade himself, because their attention happens to be fixed on him at the moment ; and the behaviour is thus a blunder of the helping instinct.[2] Another explanation which might be suggested is as follows. The presence of an injured animal with the herd is a fact which yields a disturbance to the gregarious instinct ; and in the perception of the other members of the herd it is moreover a continuously disturbing factor. On the part of the other

---

[1] Köhler, *Mentality of Apes*, 293-5.
[2] Hudson, *Naturalist in La Plata*, 339-45.

members therefore there arises an excitement, which includes an impulse to restore the normal condition of the herd. The destruction of the unfit member, while the main body of the herd survives, is certainly one way in which the disturbing factor is once for all eliminated and the herd as a whole restored almost to its usual condition ; and it is possible that in the course of the racial history of some species this mode of working off the excitement caused by the perception of a wounded comrade may have become hereditary. Cattle are certainly not capable of such highly developed behaviour as would be involved in direct assistance to the wounded. It seems very probable therefore that the differences in the extent to which gregarious animals assist their comrades may be ascribed partly to intellectual differences, i.e. differences in the capacity to realize the need of the comrade and in the insight into cause and effect necessary to see the means of assistance ; and partly also to the competition of other instincts. Wolves usually turn on an injured member of the pack and devour him at once. No doubt they are innately organized so that the perception of blood provokes at once fierce appetite, mastering all other impulses. The gregarious impulse, as indeed is obvious, as soon as it leads to a concern for the lives of others may come into conflict with other instincts, in the main those leading to individual self-preservation. Hence the possibility of great variety of response in different species, and at different times in the same species.

In addition to assistance given to comrades when in need the gregarious instinct involves as a consequence another form of conduct which is at least partly altruistic, namely, co-operation towards a common end. Many animals hunt co-operatively, e.g. wolves, and wild dogs ; and pelicans and other fishing birds form a line or half-circle so as to drive fish into the shore. Doubtless there may be in some of these cases insight into the fact that results are obtained which could not be obtained individually, and that thus the individual is benefited by the co-operation. Intelligent foresight of this character seems to be shown in some of the elaborate stratagems which are used by wolves in decoying prey.[1] But it is difficult to see how ideas involving so much foresight could have been the origin of co-operative hunting. Co-operative hunting must in its origin have been due to the fact that the companionship was mutually pleasing to the animals engaged. A dog enjoys hunting better with a companion, as we can see, and it is a common thing for a dog to go some little distance to a neighbour and invite him, deliberately as it would seem, to share his expedition. Some sort of organization grew up after the joint activity was established and common. Any form of organization means that the individuals subordinate, at least for the time being, their own appetites and impulses to the common end ; and this temporary subordination must arise, in part at least, because the individual feels some satisfaction in working with his herd and forwarding the ends of the herd as a whole. Another form of co-operative activity very common in gregarious species which are exposed to attack from enemies is the posting of sentries. A certain amount of system sometimes appears in this. The following is an observation of the changing of sentries in flocks of wild geese. " The sentinel may be approached by one of the flock and touched, after which it lowers its head and begins to feed, while the relief bird assumes the watching position—or it may, as has also been seen, force another bird to take its place by dealing it a hard peck."[2] We cannot be sure of the stages by which this amount of system has grown up. It seems however plain that, as it exists, it means that the sentinel when he first undertakes the job, and while he acts, must be repressing his own impulse to feed ; and the motive under which he does this can only be the satisfaction he obtains in the awareness that the flock in general is secured against

---

[1] Interesting examples are given by Schneider, *Der Tierische Wille*, 332–5.

[2] Finn, *Bird Behaviour*, 279.

danger. That is to say, the behaviour must include some concern for the safety of the flock as a unitary whole.

That man is a gregarious animal need hardly be insisted on. Köhler says that the chimpanzee kept in solitude is not a real chimpanzee at all.[1] And we can hardly doubt that man's gregariousness derives in direct line from some ape-like ancestor. If we look back at the account given previously of early altruistic actions of children in protecting and assisting other living things, and of their pleasure in co-operation, we shall, I think, conclude with some plausibility that such behaviour is connected with man's primitive gregariousness. These forms of conduct lead up to the fraternal type of sentiment, which thus would seem to be the most fundamental and widely spread type of love. We find that there are some writers who maintain that gregariousness in man is of a secondary character. As instances of the imperfectly social nature of man Carveth Read quotes, " the hypocrite, the criminal, the vagrant, the contra-suggestible, the hermit, the sceptic, the saint ", and points to the desire of solitude which is a normal characteristic of man.[2] Tansley also considers that the gregarious habit has a secondary origin, and that hence its main operation in the societies of to-day is to regulate and control the positive impulses derived from the self-preservative instincts.[3] The fact surely is that always from the first there is the possibility that an impulse pointing towards the maintenance of other life may conflict with the needs of individual self-preservation. Even in animal societies this may mean varieties and discrepancies in the sort of response made in the same species to similar situations, though only in man is there possibility of the awareness of conflict and deliberate hesitation between alternatives. All this has been pointed out already. To a very large extent no doubt gregariousness does act to regulate the self-preservative instincts, inasmuch as self-preservation

[1] *Mentality of Apes*, 293.   [2] C. Read, *Origin of Man*, 35.
[3] Tansley, *The New Psychology*, 201-4.

is the primary impulse of living things. But this does not prove that gregariousness and the impulse to fellowship have not their roots also very deep, not only in human, but also in animal nature. Drever is indeed of opinion that there is something primordial about the whole experience involved in the operation of this instinct, and says that, if the biologist should come to the conclusion that it is very ancient, the psychologist could not refuse him full support.[1] Complete solitude does indeed seem to have a depressing effect on the human mind which may be almost overwhelming. It is possible that no crucial test on this point has ever been made. Alexander Selkirk is described as having, during the first months of his solitude on Juan Fernandez, fallen into utter despair, and as having been saved from suicide only by turning to thoughts of religion. Thereafter he recovered his mental balance. But it may be observed that he was in continual contact with animal life, both as hunter, and as companion to the cats and goats which he tamed and with which he associated.[2] Undoubtedly there is a strong desire for intervals of solitude on the part of certain minds, principally those of advanced intellectual type. They feel the need to collect themselves and think their own thoughts, free from the insistent claim on the attention made by the presence of others. Dostoievsky, after his experience of Siberian captivity, wrote of " the poignant and terrible suffering which there is in never being alone, even for an instant, during ten years ".[3] Yet on the other hand one may surmise that among the working classes of our large cities there must be many who pass long periods of their lives without ever being quite alone ; and we do not hear a similar complaint. On the whole, and for the great majority of men, one may well believe that this need of occasional solitude does not possess the same primitive force and urgency as would

---

[1] Drever, *Instinct in Man*, 185.
[2] See *Life of Alexander Selkirk*, by J. Howell (1829).
[3] *Souvenirs de la Maison des Morts*, Part I, chap. 1.

exist in the passionate desire for a fellow human face on the part of one compelled to be solitary. The impulse towards companionship must also be more fundamental than that towards mating and parenthood. Human beings do exist without mating and parenthood, and though the results for the mind may sometimes be unfortunate, as the psycho-analysts have shown, yet often the deprivation does not appear to make much difference. On the other hand, life without any companionship at all will always have an overwhelming effect. The human being in complete solitude is likely to be profoundly affected in all his mental life.

There is a distinction to be drawn between the love of companionship and altruism ; but I am inclined to think it is not always quite accurately stated. The distinction is sometimes spoken of as though it were between an impulse to one's own pleasure, and one directed outwards to the good of others. A statement of this kind overlooks the fact that an instinct, such as the gregarious, tends by its original nature to look outwards. It is directed towards the maintenance or restoration of an objective situation. Success is accompanied by pleasure, and it is possible for man at a certain stage of intellectual development, to some extent though never completely, to regard the pleasantness of success in isolation, and to make it an end of action. This applies to other instincts as well as the gregarious, and it is a subject to be discussed later on more general lines. It has no direct relation to the distinction between a " selfish " love of society and altruism. The distinction to be drawn here is, as I conceive it, as follows. There is in the first place a side of the gregarious instinct which involves rather a passive self-surrender than active self-devotion. The agent gives himself to the companionship of others as affording comfort and protection, and a relief from isolation. In this self-surrender there may be a certain loss of the sense of individuality. The mental state of the agent may become less alert and vigorous than when he relies on himself alone. He sinks into the crowd. He also tends to become submissive towards his herd and peculiarly liable to follow any suggestion of action which may be given by it. This is decidedly exemplified in the close dependence on his society which we see in the savage. " With them ", as written of the Marquesas natives, " there hardly appeared to be any difference of opinion on any subject whatever. . . . They showed this spirit of unanimity in every action of life ; everything was done in concert and good fellow-ship ".[1] There are forms of the gregarious instinct in which this passive element is relatively more prominent. But an active self-giving to the interests of others is the normal continuation and completion of the passive self-surrender. The one passes into the other by a natural transition. "To the savage the whole gens is the individual, and he is full of regard for it. Strike the gens anywhere and every member of it considers himself struck, and the whole body corporate rises up in arms against the striker."[2] The reason why at some stages of development gregarious animals show indifference to the fortune of their comrades must be ascribed in the main to difference of intellectual capacity, to inability to realize the meaning of the expressive signs given by others, and lack of insight into the means necessary to assist. This is probably the case with the Damaraland ox, which Dalton gives as his example of passive gregariousness. It is probably for the same reason that children often appear as unfeeling or cruel. The child too is passing gradually during his development from the earliest stage, in which the presence of others is solely a comfort and a relief from isolation, to the later stages in which his interest in others is active. We saw this when dealing with the filial and fraternal relationships. We must seek for a different reason why, at a more advanced stage of in-tellectual development, we find individual persons, who

---

[1] Melville, *Typee*, quoted by Westermarck, *Origin and Development of Moral Ideas*, I, 113.

[2] Fison and Howitt, *Kamilaroi and Kurnai*, quoted by Westermarck, op. cit., I, 114.

take a great pleasure in society, but yet would not make any sacrifice in order to assist their fellows when in need. The reason here must be mainly the competition of other instinctive impulses. These persons accept the companionship of others and enjoy it for its own sake, as long as things go smoothly. But as soon as a situation arises in which a choice is necessary between attaining the end of some other instinct, which affects the individual himself only, and attaining the end of the gregarious instinct by means of assistance given to others, then it is the former which carries the day. It is thus a question of the relative strength of the instincts involved, and this in actual cases is likely to be very largely determined by habits and tendencies to action formed from early childhood. As a matter of fact we do, I think, find that the type of character mentioned above is somewhat exceptional. As a general rule sociability goes with some amount of unselfish kindliness, and the solitary tends to be self-centred, wrapped up in his own interests.

It becomes necessary here to describe in more detail than hitherto the nature of sympathy and its relation to the altruistic impulses. The question of the knowledge of other minds is one which has often been felt to give difficulty. The simplest way to put the matter seems to me this. We distinguish an external body as living by reason chiefly of the quality of its movements, which show the same temporal form as our own. In virtue of this character it is classed with the living as distinguished from the inanimate, the distinction being at first only intuitive and practical, later explicit and conscious. At the same time we distinguish the movements of the external body from those of our own body, chiefly because we experience our own movements as resulting directly from our felt needs and impulses, whereas the movements of the external body do not issue directly from our needs, and are indeed frequently experienced as directly impeding or conflicting with them. We described this somewhat more fully in dealing with the growth of self-assertion. The gregarious instinct presupposes that this amount of discrimination is possible, i.e. that there is awareness of external life, and of the difference of it from the inanimate ; for the situation which it seeks is the presence of others of the same species, living and in normal vigour. It presupposes also of course that life and mind or consciousness go together. So far as we can tell however this awareness, if it existed by itself without any other factor, would only be from the outside, as a purely cognitive matter. Through sympathy there is added to it another element, a vividness of realization of the external life, which would presumably otherwise be absent. Sympathy in its primitive form is closely connected with automatic or involuntary imitation. When movements, attitudes, or sounds produced by others are perceived, the percipient tends in such imitation to produce similar movements, attitudes, or sounds himself. The process is one similar to that reproduction through association which has a purely physiological and unconscious basis. When I perceive another perform an action, some of the same nervous tracts are activated, and in the same form, as when a similar action was carried out by myself. This partial excitation tends to pass by an automatic process into the excitation of the same whole as previously, and in the same form, provided that there are no sufficient inhibiting causes.[1] It is thus that the sight of others yawning or laughing gives a strong suggestion which frequently leads to our yawning or laughing ourselves, and in general the idea of any movement tends in the absence of inhibiting factors to pass into the actual movement. When however an agent has produced an external action or gesture, he finds himself tending to feel mentally too the emotion which is associated with that sort of movement. By emotion here we must be understood to mean the total mental state denominated by such descriptions as anger, fear, joy, etc., i.e. including feeling,

---

[1] It is admitted that this is a somewhat brief and perfunctory statement on the question of imitation, on which there is at present very little general agreement.

conative impulse, and organic sensations. If through the contagion of others' laughter we begin to laugh, though without knowing the cause, we shall begin to feel a mood of general cheerfulness and contentment, which may be described as " objectless ". The first result of the sympathetic induction is thus a state of objectless emotion, in which there is present at the same time an awareness that such emotion has been induced by the example of another living body. There are in the animal world, and perhaps also in ourselves, a certain number of inherited adaptations of nervous structure which bring it about that the perception of the signs of emotion in others immediately induces the same emotion in the percipient. Thus it is established that the heard sound of the fear note uttered by an adult bird in many cases induces fear in the young bird prior to any experience. Nestlings crouch down in the nest with all the signs of fear as soon as the warning note is heard, and, even before emerging from the shell, the young bird seems to respond similarly to the fear note.[1] Such adaptations must have become gradually established in the course of racial history. It is possible that some similar inherited dispositions in the form of a particular response to particular sorts of cries (e.g. those of fear or anger) may exist in the human race. It is also possible that there may be some inherited imitations, that is to say cases in which an inherited nervous mechanism brings it about that the perception of movement of a certain form induces a response in movement of a similar form. But it is all somewhat doubtful. In any case it is not possible to believe that the sympathetic induction of the many varied forms of emotion and feeling, which we observe in ordinary life, can be due to causes of this sort. The number of special nervous connections required would be impossibly large. For the most part in the human race sympathy in this, its simplest form, must arise because the signs of an emotion in another tend to induce a similar emotion in the beholder through

[1] Hudson, *Naturalist in La Plata*, 90.

the medium of the suggestion (even if only incipient) of the production of similar movements, attitudes, or sounds. In dealing with our present subject, we are concerned with the sympathetic induction of unpleasant feeling in its various forms. A person in a state of depression, as the result of either mental or bodily causes, will betray the same by his attitudes and gestures and perhaps by the utterance of sounds. The perception of these signs may induce an imitative reproduction on the part of an onlooker, and therewith the latter may experience a tendency to the same sort of depression. What is induced in this manner would be a bodily depression ; for it is only the external bodily signs of suffering which can be thus imitated. It is however obvious that the bodily depression thus induced is in most cases likely to be only a very pale copy or reflection of the original, for as a rule the external signs of suffering of themselves cannot induce any serious bodily disturbance, and often they have no very direct relation to the facts of the bodily disturbance. There are certain cases in which the external signs bear a very close relation to the internal bodily disturbance ; and here sympathetic induction may have a powerful effect ; as when the perception of another retching creates or increases a tendency to vomit on the part of an onlooker. But this is exceptional. For the most part suffering thus induced sympathetically is a slight affair. What converts it into something stronger and more important in conduct is a further mental process. The perception of the external signs of suffering in another leads, or may lead, by an associative process in the mind of the onlooker, to an ideal reconstruction of the total situation in which the sufferer stands. The attitudes and expressions of the sufferer may stir recollections in the onlooker of his own unpleasant experiences in the past, physical or mental. Verbal description is of course the way in which the experiences of one person can be most completely communicated to another. But it is not necessary in order to produce an ideal reconstruction on the part of the onlooker. The suggestion given by the movements, bringing about the tendency to imitation already described, may be enough to give an idea of the total mental state of the sufferer. It is in this manner that there is reached the fully developed form which sympathy takes, namely the experiencing by one person of feelings similar to those experienced by another, as a result of an idea of the total situation in which the latter stands, including both his cognitions and his strivings in response to them, there being at the same time an awareness of the separate existence of the other. Such sympathetic feelings certainly may reach a somewhat high degree of intensity. A vivid realization of the position of another who has suffered a bereavement may, by causing us to " act out " the situation fully, put us for the time being ideally in the position of a bereaved person, and make us feel extremely sad. But, as has not unfrequently been pointed out by other writers, this experience does not in itself yield an effective impulse towards the sort of action usually termed unselfish. It is no doubt possible to terminate the unpleasant experience due to the contagion of another's melancholy by endeavouring to assist or comfort him. But the more direct and effective way would be to remove from his neighbourhood or to adopt some other means of distracting our attention. If we are contagiously affected by the presence of another in some way which is displeasing to us, that is indeed the obvious way of terminating the situation. Even if, moreover, we should try to assist another for this reason, we should be treating him merely as a means to secure a pleasant state of mind for ourselves. The action would terminate on our situation, not on his. On the other hand there is yielded by the gregarious instinct, as we have described it, an impulse which looks outwards and terminates on the objective situation of another ; and it is only here that actually unselfish conduct is to be found. The rôle played by sympathy herein will be as follows. Given the fact that there exists already this instinct towards the well-being of our fellows, then a fuller " content " and body is given to that instinct by the tendency to reconstruct and " act out " in ourselves their experiences. We shall be able to realize more fully the nature of the conscious life of others and to enter more into their feelings, and the impulse to relieve them or to forward their interests will be able to adjust itself more closely to their needs. There being two factors presupposed, as we said at the beginning of this discussion, in the gregarious instinct, namely, awareness of the distinction of life from the inanimate and awareness of the distinction of other life from our own, it is through sympathy that there is added to this awareness of other life a vivid and detailed realization and a glow of feeling which would not otherwise exist. It will be obvious also that the altruistic impulses will be limited by the capacity for sympathetic realization. One cannot interpret signs of feeling if such signs are completely different to those which one carries out oneself ; nor can one put oneself in the place of a person experiencing any emotion, unless one is capable of experiencing something similar. Moreover, given the fact that we may become aware by means of sympathy that another is suffering, then it is in virtue of the original altruistic impulse that it becomes difficult to distract the attention from him, that the idea of his suffering is an insistent one, pointing in the direction of affording relief if possible. Thus the gregarious instinct without sympathy would be almost blind ; sympathy is its necessary tool ; while at the same time sympathy without the altruistic impulse would have no driving force as a motive.

There is, as we may believe appears from the foregoing, an original impulse which leads man to count himself in as a member with a larger body of his kind and to feel an interest in maintaining the existence of that group as a whole and the vital activity of its members. It is an original need, which prevents man from being self-sufficient to himself, takes him out of the interest of individual self-maintenance, and causes him to find a satisfaction in a self-giving to the interests of this larger whole. As H. G. Wells has put it, there is a desire to partake, towards a way out of ourselves, a breaking down of our individual separation, and only so do we find " salvation ".[1] This is a primary and underived fact of our nature. Indeed poets and preachers have many times insisted that there is in man this " will to love ". " Only that soul is happy which loves ", wrote Goethe. We do not rest content with a merely passive unity. Unless there is some active forwarding of the lives or well-being of those outside us, complete satisfaction of the impulse is hardly attained, nor, it should be added, is complete satisfaction attained unless there is some form of recipro-cation or recognition of the devotion. For otherwise the unity is incomplete and one-sided.

But the above obviously is not true of man only *qua* gregarious animal. If we look at the various forms of family affection, as we have described them, we shall see that in each there appears a form of the same impulse to self-giving. In the beginning the individual life is separ-ated off as a detached portion of other life ; and it still seems at first to feel the need of close union with other life, and perhaps preferably with that from which it was derived. Gradually a separate consciousness is developed. Though the gregarious instinct is effective in certain forms, i.e. in the impulse to help and co-operate with comrades, it is true to say that, up to the time of puberty, the main line of development is that of the individual as a separate self-seeking and self-assertive unit. In the reproductive series there is a certain breaking down of this individual self-sufficiency. The need is primarily to give oneself to the interests of those particular lives with which in reproduction there is a particular bond of unity ; it is with them that unity is primarily felt, and towards them primarily that there arises tender emotion. But we may also perhaps speak in some sense of a return to a unity with that original stream of life from which the individual

---

[1] H. G. Wells, *First and Last Things*, Book II, § 8. Book IV, § 2.

o

was derived. In conjugation and parenthood there must be some sense of individual insufficiency, of the necessity of union with other life in order to forward the stream of life, and so of a certain kinship with the general body of life. It has often been said that in these relations are found the first stepping-stones leading men to wider interests, though at first they may seem to be narrowing in their effect. Bergson said that it is the tendency to reproduction which everywhere opposes that to individuality.[1] Höffding writes : " In the instincts named above [those connected with reproduction] we have the helping hands which from the first lead men to something beyond themselves, and bring them into relations where the educative laws of association may operate."[2] And Rabindranath Tagore says : " It very often happens that our love for our children, our friends, or other loved ones debars us from the further realization of our soul. It enlarges our scope of consciousness no doubt, yet it sets a limit to its freest expansion. Nevertheless it is the first step, and all the wonder lies in this first step itself. It shows to us the true nature of our soul. From it we know for certain that our highest joy is in the losing of our egoistic self and in the uniting with others."[3]

We believe that from the foregoing it appears that in parental love we have, not an instinct quite separate from the gregarious instinct, but another form of an impulse which includes and is wider than both.

We should not wish to deny that in the development of the altruistic impulses natural selection has played some part. Parental tenderness and protection have of course in the animal world been of great value for survival ; and so have subordination and mutual helpfulness within the tribal group. These tendencies may well have owed some part of their development and increase to the effect of an

---

[1] Bergson, *Creative Evolution*, 14.
[2] Höffding, *Outlines of Psychology*, 251.
[3] R. Tagore, *Sadhana*, 29.
We may compare McDougall, *Group Mind*, 81-4, where he emphasizes the need of family affection as the root of wider sentiments.

inter-group struggle for existence, if we assume that the
germ of them has always existed as part of the original
nature of living beings. The course of development may
then be surmised to have been somewhat as follows.
Originally associations of animals arose because the
members of one family or brood remained together as
they grew up, provided the conditions of food supply
permitted. There was no reason for them to separate ;
and in the association there was afforded some satisfaction
of a need which had always existed in a germinal form,
the need to live and act in union with a larger body
of life. In other species the conditions of food supply
compelled separation and individual self-maintenance.
Animals of those species which remained together tended
to act together, and organization with partial subordination of the individual to the group began to appear. Such
group-organization and the spirit of devotion to the group
were often advantageous in the struggle for existence, at
first with the forces of nature, and later with other groups.
Natural selection therefore favoured these characters ;
but at first in the form of the limited group spirit, in
virtue of which devotion was felt exclusively to one's own
group, with as its obverse a feeling of hostility to other
groups. One factor in the gregarious instinct was, as
we have shown, an identification of the self with the group ;
and this primarily meant a will to the increase of the power
of one's own group as against that of other groups.
These results are however only incidental to the struggle
for existence between groups, and do not spring from the
essence of the gregarious instinct, as a will to give the
self to the interests of a larger whole. Two sets of causes
have so far as we can see led to the limits imposed by this
narrower group spirit being transcended. (1) The inter-
group struggle has itself tended to cease, partly because
of forcible amalgamations through conquest, partly
because improved methods enable food supply to be more
easily obtained from nature, while at the same time there
is a tendency in highly civilized people for the rate of

increase of population to diminish. (2) Various causes have led to a clearer intellectual recognition of our kinship with the rest of humanity, and indeed with the rest of the living universe. Among these causes the most important has been the increased knowledge of the various races by each other, due to increased ease of communication and spread of education. Thus the range of imaginative sympathy has been greatly extended. Given these factors, there is no reason to prevent a sentiment of devotion being conceived to the widest whole to which a man is capable of thinking of himself as belonging.

We may speak of such an extension as naturally following from the original character of the impulse, provided that there is the intellectual capacity to conceive of humanity or life as a whole. It would be the natural, but not perhaps the inevitable or necessary, result. For the development has in part, it cannot be denied, been dependent on the extraneous or incidental fact that the severity of competition between groups has diminished. It is not easy to forecast what may be the result if at some future time the increase of the world's population were to bring about great pressure on the world's possible food supply.

> Warless ? when her tens are thousands, and her thousands millions, then
> All her harvest all too narrow—who can fancy warless men ?

Tennyson wrote in " Locksley Hall Sixty Years After ". But into such speculations we need hardly go further here.

We spoke above of a " return " in the relations of conjugation and parenthood to that original unity from which the individual life was derived. It must be obvious that the unity to which a return is made is very different from the original unity. In the meantime selfhood has been developed ; and it does not appear that, in fact, in love there is any fusing of the bounds of personality, such as to lead to a lowering of the level of the conscious life. There is, it is true, a lessened self-consciousness, if that term is used in one of its common meanings. In terming anyone self-conscious we often mean that he thinks much of what others may be thinking of him ; and it is usually implied also that there is a certain amount of concentration on the individual interests and ends, and little thought of those of others.   There will of course be a loss of self-consciousness in this sense, inasmuch as in love the agent is concentrating directly on the existence and interests of others.   There will be a sympathetic entering into the conscious life and activities of the beloved. But through this, perhaps in the background of consciousness, there will persist a sense of the separate existence of the self, and of the fact that there is a giving of the self without its being absorbed.   The consciousness is of the self as giving and protecting.   So that love is to be experienced, not as entirely selfless, but as a continuous self-giving ; not necessarily expressed in continuous acts of service, but perhaps in a constant protective attitude, in which there may always be near the surface of the conscious mental stream that fear of harm to the beloved, which we found expressed in Heine's well-known poem.

The same may be said to be true where the altruistic impulse is expressed in some form of self-devotion to a wider whole than that of the family.   One may surmise that for the gregarious animal, when with his herd, the satisfaction of the gregarious instinct yields as a rule nothing but a permanent background of comfort to the mental life.   He is only conscious of the instinct when it is disturbed in some way.   Then there is strong conscious effort towards the restoration of the normal situation. Apart from this the situation would be one with which the animal remains passively content, and the level of mental activity and of consciousness would be somewhat lower than with a solitary animal, compelled to rely on itself entirely for safety and sustenance.   With man too no doubt the accustomed society of others will often appear as nothing but a passively accepted fact, yielding a background of comfort to the mental life.   There are however in the social life of man many activities in the service of the community which can be experienced as a continuous self-giving to the interests of a larger whole. Moreover in any co-operative work which involves division of labour and therefore some adjustment to other selves, differing more or less in capacities and qualities from the agent, the sense of individual personality on the part of the latter must be increased rather than diminished by the contrast. Hence the level of consciousness may remain a high one.

If we compare the relation to others in altruistic action with that in competition and conflict, we shall see that the latter involves relatively, no doubt, a very intense, but at the same time a somewhat narrow, form of self-feeling. The interest in others is confined to the one point in respect of which there is conflict. The attention is only concentrated on the opponent in order to get the best of him in that one point. Hence the agent's own consciousness of himself tends also to be narrowed to the one point at which he is in conflict with another. But in the going out of the self in order to take an interest or delight in the life of others, there is involved a sense of self-enlargement which seems to have two grounds, firstly in the fact that the relation is one of participation instead of opposition, secondly in the fact that interest is felt in the *whole* of the personality of others instead of being narrowed to one point. This is not to make any pronouncement on final values, or to say that a reconciliation is thus to be found between "egoism" and "altruism". It may still be the case that a conflict will occur between the impulses of love to others and other instincts, such as ambition or the pursuit of knowledge ; and we make no statement as to which end ultimately possesses the higher value. All that is asserted here is that in the self-giving of love there is a form of experience, which for a highly conscious being is one possessing a peculiar value of its own, and not involving any lowering of the level of the conscious life.

The comparison made above is between altruism and

egoism as involving competition with others, not between altruism and that form of conduct known as "pure" cruelty. Cruelty in its purest form is a seeking of the sense of power through hurt inflicted on others; it is in the fact that the agent knows the others to be suffering consciously that the sense of power is sought. It is no doubt the fact that the agent does in this way attain a very intense form of self-feeling. The reason why men as a rule regard such pure cruelty with intense horror and aversion is surely just this: that it is felt to be a direct contradiction and reversal of the impulses of love and tender emotion, and that the satisfaction of these latter impulses is felt to possess a peculiar value of its own. If we inflict injury on another as an incident of the fact that both are competing for the same object, there is a relation of contrariety between egoistic and altruistic impulses; but we feel that it is more or less accidental. To take pleasure in the very fact of inflicting suffering on another is felt as directly contradicting and outraging our impulses to love and tenderness. Hence the apparently immediate and instinctive repulsion which the normal man feels at the idea of such action. Its immediate character is surely a testimony to the strength of the appeal which love makes to us. For it at once outweighs any appeal which the heightened sense of power in cruelty might make. Just as there is a peculiar pleasure in the satisfaction of the impulse to altruistic love, so it would seem there is a peculiar unpleasure, for the normal man, in the experience of having failed to satisfy it or contradict it. Without entering on questions of moral philosophy, we may assert that at least one element in remorse is the sense that, by inflicting injury on a member of one's community, one has contradicted the impulse of altruistic love and thereby brought about a separation of the self from the community to which it belongs. Hence a feeling of conflict or division within the self; for the altruistic impulses still persist and yet are felt to have been thwarted of reaching their due expression.

It is perhaps possible to connect the impulse of which we have spoken, that towards self-giving to a larger whole, with the mystic experience, as it is described for us by many who have had it personally. Of such descriptions we may quote Tennyson's : " This (a kind of waking trance) has come upon me through repeating my own name to myself silently, till all at once, as it were out of the intensity of the consciousness of individuality, individuality itself seemed to dissolve and fade away into boundless being, and this not a confused state but the clearest, the surest of the surest, utterly beyond words—where death was an almost laughable impossibility—the loss of personality (if so it were) seeming no extinction, but the only true life. . . . It is no nebulous ecstasy, but a state of transcendent wonder, associated with absolute clearness of mind."[1] And this from the Upanishads : " Like as a falcon or an eagle tiring after wide circuits in the windy spaces of heaven foldeth his wings and droppeth to quiet cover, so urgeth the spirit towards that state whose repose no desire troubleth nor delusion entereth. That is its true being, from yearnings, from evil and from fear delivered. Like unto a man in the embrace of a beloved wife, unaware of things without or things within, is the spirit that is embraced by the all-discerning self. This one second is an ocean, free from duality, this, O King ! is the world of Brahman. . . . This is his highest goal, this his dearest success, this his greatest world, and this his supreme rapture."[2] It is not difficult to draw the parallel between these states of mind and those which we have been dealing with. In each sort of case it may be said there is a self-surrender without loss of consciousness or degradation of its level. Though many of the mystics apparently assert the loss of self-consciousness, yet it is doubtful in what sense this is to be taken, and there is no doubt that what they describe is a very vivid form of conscious experience. If there is any truth in this com-

---

[1] Quoted by James, *Varieties of Religious Experience*, 384.
[2] Quoted by Jung, *Psychological Types*, 246.

parison, we should be able to say that the awareness of unity with a larger whole, which is only attained by the ordinary mind in a partial form through concrete acts in the service of other life, can be attained directly and in a more complete form by some exceptional minds through direct willing. It is a further question whether the larger whole, with which the individual feels himself to be in union, has objective existence, in its widest form as universal mind or spirit. James held that " in the fact that the conscious person is continuous with a wider self through which saving experiences come, we have a positive content of religious experience, which is literally and objectively true as far as it goes ".[1] It is beyond the scope of a psychological treatise to attempt to deal with this question, as psychology starts from the standpoint of individual mind only. We are, I think, justified from the point of view of psychology in stating how things appear to the individual mind, without going on to determine how or in what sense the larger self, with which it feels as though it were continuous, possesses objective existence.

[1] James, *Varieties of Religious Experience*, 515.

CHAPTER VI

SUMMARY AND CLASSIFICATION OF THE HUMAN INSTINCTS

WE may now attempt to give a summary and classification of the instinctive equipment of man. The fundamental fact with which we start is the self-maintaining bodily process, of which the chief part is the function of nutrition. In the course of racial history, as the result of the effort to maintain this process in the face of impediments of various kinds or in face of changed external circumstances, there have appeared a number of auxiliary tendencies, which in the course of time have become fixed by heredity and appear as separate instincts. Such are appetitions towards or aversions from specific sorts of objects, tendencies towards construction, towards acquisition and storage, towards pursuit and hunting for its own sake, and towards periodical change of abode. The development even of the intellectual faculties must have been due at first to the same causes. A cognitive element is of course a necessary part of all mental life. But the development and elaboration of the cognitive powers must have been in its earliest stages due to the advantages which intellectual power gave in the struggle to maintain the bodily process and principally that of nutrition. When any such separate tendency becomes established as an inherited instinct, it acquires thereby a certain independence. There will often arise an urge to fulfil it apart from the existence of the nutritive needs which it originally subserved. There will be a pleasantness moreover attaching to such independent exercise. Given that any bodily or mental capacity has become established and hereditary, its exercise as it matures will be pleasant for itself. There are two forms of reaction, i.e. fear and anger, which are subsidiary to the vital self-maintaining process in a sense different to that just mentioned. Those mentioned in the preceding paragraph are specific tendencies in relation to specific external circumstances. Fear and anger are more generalized forms of reaction, taking place in response to any sort of interference with the vital process, or the activities subsidiary thereto. Whenever there is any such interference, fear or anger, according to circumstances, is likely to arise. Both involve in a rudimentary form an attitude of a self. Fear is especially a prospective mental activity. It is the reaction in relation to a depressed or obstructed state of vital activity, while that depression or obstruction is looked forward to as likely to get worse, and it carries with it a conative effort to escape from the cause of the harm and thus resume the normal vital course. Anger is a form of reaction, which involves a stronger self-assertion ; in it the mind turns on the cause of the obstruction with an effort to destroy or expel it. Both tendencies are thus originally general, being a further continuation of that series of which unpleasure is the starting point. But it is possible also for both to become established as specific inherited tendencies in relation to particular objects or sets of circumstances. It is possible for specific objects which in the past history of the race have caused fear or anger now to arouse these tendencies in advance of any actual harm caused. There has been a good deal of discussion as to what these specific angers or fears are in the animal world, and it is true that in some cases fears, which have been thought to be specific and hereditary, have been shown to be due to the teaching or example of adult companions.[1] But there can be no doubt that there are some such inherited specific tendencies. For example, I think any one who has observed the peculiar attitude of ordinary domestic cattle towards a dog can have no doubt that here there is an inherited blend of anger and

[1] See Hudson, *Naturalist in La Plata*, chap. 5.

fear towards the descendant of a species which was a
danger in the past history of the race.[1] In man it is very
doubtful whether there are any inherited tendencies of
either fear or anger towards specific objects, such as
animals. As the result of experiments on babies Watson
has concluded that there is no instinctive fear of animals,
and believes that the only fears elicited from babies are
when the accustomed material support is suddenly withdrawn, and when sudden loud sounds are heard.[2] These
results agree well enough with the view that fear is a
reaction to which the mind is innately predisposed as
part of the constant *nisus* to maintain the normal vital
process. Fear always, we may say, lies somewhat near
the surface of the mental life, ready to be called out by
any sudden disturbance ; and it may well be that the
human mind is so organized by heredity that, apart from
and prior to experience of harm, it responds with fear to
the two kinds of disturbance mentioned, namely loud
noises and withdrawal of support. Of course with experience of bodily harm other forms of fear soon appear in
the growing child. We must however also mention another
form in which it is possible to speak of inherited anger
and fear. The attitude of either fear or anger may become
fixed in a species in such a way that its individual members
are in general predisposed to one of these forms of reaction in response to any stimulus, and in particular to any
sort of opposition. Some species of animals, and also
perhaps some races of men, are innately timid, and others
innately irritable and pugnacious. The circumstances
of their development together with accidental variations
must, as we may believe, have led to their reactions
becoming organized in one or other of these patterns.

At a certain stage of evolution, as the result of selection
in the struggle for existence, there appears an animal with
the intellectual capacity to plan ahead for its future

[1] I have seen a cow with a calf make a sudden fierce charge on a dog,
while paying no attention to human beings near at hand.
[2] Watson, *Psychology from the Standpoint of a Behaviourist*, 219–21
and 222–6.

and to remember its own past in order to guide these plans, and so with some idea, rudimentary though it may be at first, of itself as a continuing existence and of other selves as contrasted with or opposing it. As soon as this stage has been reached, it becomes possible for there to emerge from the automatically self-maintaining vital process a will for the preservation of the individual self and a conscious aversion to its extinction by death. From the first however, as we hope to have shown, this will for the preservation of the individual self tends to pass into a will to self-maximation, or to power. Power becomes a separate object of pursuit, dominance over other living beings or external nature being sought for its own sake. The satisfaction of the will to power then also enters as an element into the satisfaction of a number of other instincts, originally subsidiary to self-preservation, and adds to them an additional value. It enters thus into the exercise of the inborn, bodily and mental, capacities, into the exercise of man's cognitive faculties, making out of them an impulse which leads towards the formation of the ordered world of knowledge, into the constructive, acquisitive, and hunting instincts, and into the combative instinct in the case of those species innately predisposed to anger. Indeed for a highly conscious self the elation going with the sense of power yields almost the whole of the value which the satisfaction of these instincts possesses. As compared with the bodily needs and the instincts subsidiary to self-preservation, we find there comes into existence a constant tendency to regard the will to self-maximation as " higher " in kind, as possessing a superior sort of value. We shall hope later to deal with this question further. But we may give here two valid reasons which appear to exist for the opinion stated above. In the first place mere self-preservation along the lines of already given instinct becomes soon a somewhat dull and routine affair. In the sense of power there is felt to be a movement forward to an intenser form of conscious existence, and this must naturally yield a stronger and more vivid satisfaction. In the second place, however closely the conscious self is bound up with the maintenance of the bodily sensations, it cannot be held to be *identical* with them. There is always the possibility that to a highly conscious self the bodily needs and their satisfactions, leading to the preservation of the bodily life, will appear as something imposed by the constraint of a necessary material substratum, and not appertaining to the essential nature of the self. In the sense of dominance and the feeling of elation it seems rather as though the self moved forward of itself, expressing its own nature, as though an impulse essential to it were being fulfilled. A humiliation may touch such conscious beings more nearly than the hurt of a blow, or even than the unpleasant pangs of hunger. I think the ordinary language and thought of human beings, in proportion as intellectually developed, bears witness to the fact that this distinction is actually felt.

It is obvious that fear and anger play the same safeguarding rôle in relation to the will to power that they do in relation to the bodily instincts. We look forward with fear to the possibility of this will being frustrated, and external opposition to it is met with anger.

In one of its functions the bodily process points beyond its own individual self-maintenance. Growth leads to reproduction, i.e. to the separation from the living body of portions which become other living individual bodies. It is in this function and the activities subsidiary thereto that there is a certain primary breaking down of the isolation of the individual life ; it feels itself bound to, and interested in, other life. There emerges an awareness of the individual self as forming part of a larger unity, and a need to live and act for the interests of that larger whole. This appears as a separate positive impulse in the form of love, and also it enters into life as controlling or opposing the impulses of self-preservation and self-maximation. Sometimes too it enters into other instincts as modifying them and adding to them a further element

of value, as in the case of the scientific devotion to truth.
Like the impulse to self-maximation, the impulse to self-
giving can only be considered as part of the essential
nature of mind. As such it must be contrasted with the
purely bodily activities involved in reproduction ; for
the latter are likely to appear, in as far as a high intellectual level has been reached, as something imposed by the
material substratum of life, and not as an expression
of the nature of the conscious self. In the case of the will
to power it is possible to see how it develops out of the
self-preserving effort present in all life. But within the
limits of psychology it is hardly possible to ascribe an
origin to the impulse to self-giving. It appears in its
earliest form in the care given to the offspring produced
by the individual. But this is no account of its ultimate
origin. If psychology necessarily starts from the standpoint of mind as individual and confines itself to that
standpoint, it can give no account of the ultimate origin
of this impulse, nor of the peculiar form of satisfaction
which accompanies its exercise. We seem pointed beyond
the limits of mind as individual.

Fear and anger have a relation to this impulse somewhat different from that which they have to the other
instincts. They are provoked in their ordinary form, when
by some external impediment the agent is prevented
from carrying out his wish to join himself physically
with the community of his fellows. But in regard to
the more active side of the impulse, that to self-giving
to the interests of the community, it is rather different.
No man can be prevented from the mental act of giving
himself in love, from taking delight in other life. The
shocks or frustrations to which the impulse is subjected
occur when by some external agency the vital activity
of one's fellows undergoes diminution or obstruction.
Anger or fear can be felt disinterestedly on behalf of others
in these circumstances. We fear for others or are indignant
on their behalf. Even if a man is prevented from carrying
out the external acts by which he would assist others, his

fear or anger is not experienced in the form of a reaction against a frustrated impulse of his own. His attention being concentrated in the main on the good of others, his emotional impulse will concern itself directly with them, and the fear or anger which he feels will still take a disinterested form.

We would then put forward the view that the original instinctive equipment of man is made up as follows: In the first place the self-maintaining bodily process, including growth and propagation, together with a number of activities subsidiary thereto which have been created in the course of evolution; in the second place the two impulses in which there expresses itself the nature of the spiritual element lying behind the facts of life, those to self-maximation and self-giving; and lastly fear and anger, which act as reactions safeguarding the other impulses.

It will here be as well to ask provisionally whether there is any distinction to be drawn between instincts of a " higher " and those of a " lower " level. There are two possible principles of distinction. In the first place, as the result of intellectual development there comes into existence a clearer prevision of the course of a conation and of the end towards which it tends, so that actions can be more definitely directed towards that end. There is some prevision in all instinct, as Stout has well shown. But with animals this need be nothing more than an awareness of the present situation as transitional or unsatisfactory, and a will to alter it, which has no clear foresight of the future, but moves in a certain direction, which is found satisfying as it proceeds, other directions being unsatisfying.[1] Nothing more than this need be supposed to exist even in such prolonged trains of action as propagation, nest-building, and rearing of the young by birds. With man there is a possibility of action being directed towards a clearly foreseen end. But we need not conclude that

[1] Stout, *Manual of Psychology*, chapter on " Instinct," specially pp. 355–6.

this fact in itself makes any difference to the nature of the
" urge " or " impulse " in the conation. The fact that
mental planning of a complex order may be employed
as means does not necessarily make any difference to the
conation itself. In order either to set aside a present
experience of hunger or pain, or to guard against the
possibility of such an experience occurring in the future,
it is possible that use may be made of complex intellectual
operations. But in spite of this the impulse to avoid
hunger or pain remains essentially the same.

The second possible principle of distinction relates
more to the ends of instinct rather than to the subsidiary
means. As the result of intellectual development ends
of a different order appear. Acceptance or rejection is
directed, not to a sensory fact, but towards a total perceptual situation, which includes relations. For instance,
the instinct to construct a shelter means bringing into
existence a complex perceived whole. A perceived pattern
again is, to an intellect which has reached a certain
development, either satisfactory or unsatisfactory, according as the arrangement of its parts either facilitates attention to it as a whole, or renders it difficult by confusing
and baffling attention. The satisfaction of the self-assertive impulse depends on a relation apprehended between
the self (of which the agent may be more or less clearly
conscious) and other selves or external force. With
developed intellects the formation of the most highly
generalized concepts becomes an end. The most important
of these " higher " ends arises with the formation of the
idea of a conscious self or personality. It then becomes
possible to aim at the enhancement of the conscious life
of the self in the sense of power ; and it also becomes
possible to find a satisfaction in the devotion of that
conscious self to wider interests. It might be maintained
that here again however there is no ultimate difference
in the nature of the conation involved. Even the impulses towards the highest forms of self-development
or self-devotion might be said to come to us as immediate,

P

imposed by our mental constitution, and not as a matter of individual choice. We have stated above why a higher value is usually ascribed to these impulses than to those of bodily maintenance ; and will defer the further consideration of this question for the present, dealing further first with the relation of feeling to instinct.

CHAPTER VII

THE RELATION OF FEELING TO THE INSTINCTS

WE will now ask what is the relation of feeling to the instincts as thus described and classified. That the successful fulfilment of these instincts is accompanied by pleasure and their frustration by unpleasure, seems obvious at first sight. There is however a view of life, which we often find implied in ordinary thought, to the effect that pleasure lies only in the attainment of ends, and that life is made up for the most part of wants and the efforts made towards the pleasurable moments of attainment. This view worked out thoroughly and consistently leads to the theory of the pessimistic philosophers that the normal and positive state of the mind is one of unpleasant want, that it is driven by a necessity of its nature to try and pass from the unpleasant present to a future less irksome, and that pleasure is nothing positive, but only a temporary and relative liberation from unpleasure. We find statements similar to this, which purport to be actual judgments passed on experience of life. Goethe, who if anyone might be thought to have lived a life of successful and many-sided activity, wrote as follows : " I will say nothing against the course of my existence. But at bottom it has been nothing but pain and burden, and I can affirm that, during the whole of my seventy-five years, I have not had four weeks of genuine well-being. It is but the perpetual rolling of a rock, that must be raised up again for ever."[1] I suppose a theory of this sort is implied also in Bradley's criticism of the view that there can be any ultimate goodness in a desire or volition, inasmuch as it is a state inconsistent

---

[1] Quoted by James, *Varieties of Religious Experience*, 137.

with itself, striving always to pass beyond itself, to abolish itself by the fulfilment of the desire.[1] Does a theory of the essentially conative nature of all mental life lend support to this ? We may well ask whether the contradiction is actually felt by men, whether they necessarily experience life in the form thus stated. We have seen that there are a number of instincts which mature gradually, while others, principally those connected directly with nutrition, appear in full force from the first. In those cases in which the instinct matures gradually, it often first becomes effective as a conscious motive in the form of a reaction to some unpleasant shock of disappointment. This however presupposes that the instinct itself was previously in existence in a latent or subconscious form. In the nature of things there is no reason why the maturation of an instinct such as sexual love, or the development of the bodily and intellectual capacities, should not, as we have seen, take place gradually and be experienced as pleasant throughout. The lives of the majority of adult human beings are occupied with self-maintenance and its subsidiary activities, plus the working out of the reproductive impulse. The latter involves a conative train which should normally cover many years, and which may be said to fulfil itself successfully as it is gradually worked out. Self-maintenance for many men, though not for all, means periodical trains of conative activity, the getting through to its end of some connected job ; e.g. for the farmer the completion of his harvest, for the craftsman his article turned out, for the clerk a report or an audit finished. For all it means some exercise of bodily and mental powers, even if it be monotonous, which results in the support of life. It is doubtless possible to hold that we work in order that we may eat, and that the conative trains of action, which we have mentioned, are something extraneous to the pleasurable end, which exists apart from the work which obtains it. But it is

---

[1] Bradley, *Appearance and Reality*, chapter on " Goodness," e.g. pp. 410 and 432.

also possible to hold that we do not live only in order that we may eat, we eat also that we may live, and that life consists in some exercise of the bodily powers. For most people this is some sort of work and earning ; and thus life would constitute what Stout has called a " re-entrant series ".[1] The winning of food and the other essentials of life, and their consumption, would together make up life. It is this latter view that seems to me the normal and natural. The point at which the distinction should be drawn between the pleasurable and unpleasurable seems to be rather this. Sometimes activity makes no progress ; there is no felt working out of the conative train to its end. These points of stoppage must necessarily be unpleasant in themselves, though, if not too prolonged, they may often be felt as giving additional keenness and zest to the activity. But whenever there is a certain amount of progress towards the completion, then pleasure will occur. This need not involve definite anticipations, and it would be unnecessary to think of this pleasantness as only possible for a being with sufficient intelligence to anticipate ends vividly. Take the case of the hunting animal, so far as we can judge of its state of mind. Hunting is at first probably a pleasurable activity. But after a time, when no quarry is sighted and no progress made towards success, it will begin to become unpleasant. In the act of sighting the quarry and in the process of overtaking it there is a progressive attainment, which we can assume to be pleasurable. We must, I think, distinguish this pleasure of progressive attainment from any pleasure which may be yielded by the exercise of the bodily and mental powers incidentally involved as a means. If cravings for exercise are satisfied at the same time, that will be an additional source of pleasure. But the satisfaction which comes from the successful maintenance of life is something which can be felt, even if the incidental work necessary is monotonous or some-

---

[1] Stout, *Analytic Psychology*, I, 150.

what unpleasant. And there is likely to be present that note of hope and confidence which we have described as accompanying the successful maintenance of life.

If we look at the instincts which appear later in development, we shall find the existence of conative series which may be very prolonged, such as the search for knowledge or the pursuit of power, constituting the main content of a whole life. There may also appear in the individual life sporadic and recurrent trains of activity resulting from instincts of this sort. Either these arise because some impulse, which in ordinary life is adequately and continuously satisfied and therefore exists in a latent and subconscious form, is subjected to a shock of frustration, which appears as unpleasant. Or else it may be that an instinct from time to time gradually matures until it reaches sufficient strength, as it were, to compel periodical discharge in action. An instance of the first sort would be when a man, living an incurious life in his ordinary surroundings, meets suddenly with some novel sort of fact, and this starts the impulse of curiosity, which aims at fitting the new fact into his ordered world of knowledge. It would be an instance of the second sort when a man, finding that his ordinary life does not satisfy his power impulse, feels himself impelled to find satisfaction for it in occasional competitive games and sports. In all these cases it is not the case that an unpleasant state of want or desire persists up to the moment of attaining an end, which is momentarily enjoyed as pleasant and then replaced by the drive of a further want. Even for a man who fixes his gaze on some distant goal of wealth or power, felt movement in the direction of the end must have the effect of a progressive attainment and as such be pleasurable. The pleasantness in these cases need not necessarily always exist in an acute form. It will often only be a pleasantly toned background or undercurrent to the mental life. Nor would the pleasure be likely to remain at the same level throughout. If the conative train is started by the shock of some disappointment, the initial phase will be one of unpleasure. Subsequent progress is not likely to be uniform. Checks and hindrances will be unpleasant in themselves, and inasmuch as at such times there is a damming up of the conative energy, the strength of that energy will be increased. As has been well pointed out by Stout, if the impediment is not too serious and prolonged, the pleasure of the release of energy which accompanies its removal is as a rule more than equivalent to the unpleasure of the stoppage.[1] A series of checks and releases adds to the zest of the total pursuit, inasmuch as by such means we become more fully conscious of the progress of the attainment. There are also likely to be in any prolonged train of activity subsidiary incidental actions and pieces of work, less directly concerned with the ultimate end than others. In these subsidiary actions there will be less consciousness of progress in the required direction. The moment of completion, provided that completion is possible and is realized, would naturally be that of the highest pleasure, a pleasure which need not be entirely momentary, but can spread its effects in the form of a mood over a considerable period of time.

The altruistic impulses must be regarded, in respect of the point now being considered, as rather different from the other instincts. A train of activity can be undertaken in order to maintain or forward the life of others. This train of activity will be liable to all the same variations of success or failure as any other. But provided it is undertaken in a spirit of genuine self-devotion, it is likely to be accompanied by an undercurrent of satisfaction or happiness, which is not directly affected by success or non-success.

The experiment has been made of getting a number of persons to introspect their experiences over a period of days and record how the durations of pleasure and

---

[1] See Stout, *Manual of Psychology*, 696.

unpleasure compare.[1] So far as these observations go, their result is to point to the fact that in actual ordinary experience pleasure considerably outweighs unpleasure. The average for nine observers gives the duration of pleasant states as 50·1 per cent of the total, of neutral states as 27·8, and of unpleasant states as 22·2. The greater part of life according to these observations is made up of slightly pleasant and neutral states, which together make up 66·4 per cent of the total. I imagine this coincides very much with what ordinary common sense would have anticipated. Artistic natures are usually sensitive and subject to ups and downs of feeling. Such an utterance as that quoted from Goethe may well be that of a sensitive man burdened by age at a moment of depression.

The records quoted above from Flügel reflect of course the general view that there are many states which are indifferent as between pleasure and unpleasure. This is a point at which we must look, as it would seem to follow from our general view that no mental state can be entirely neutral. For we have asserted that the stuff of the mental life is made up of conational trains of activity, and in conations and pursuits there cannot be such a thing as an indifference point ; they must at any one moment be proceeding successfully or unsuccessfully. No doubt there are many individual impressions which may appear as neutral. Many objects which we notice casually around have no apparent effect on the conative mental life and do not alter its affective character. Yet though single impressions may appear as indifferent, it may well be maintained that the main current of the mental life always has a tinge of pleasure or unpleasure.[2] Probably no one would deny this of life, in so far as it is made up of alternations of desire and satisfaction. But much of life seems to be made up of habit, and habit is often thought to

[1] Flügel in *British Journal of Psychology*, April 1925, 318, etc., see especially table on p. 328.
[2] See Höffding, *Outline of Psychology*, 288, Stout, *Analytic Psychology*, II, 288, and *Manual of Psychology*, 116–18, by whom this distinction has been made.

be neutral. Certainly habit is the great deadener of the affective life. There are many routine acts throughout the day, which we do almost mechanically, and often think of as indifferent. But if the matter is looked at more closely I think it is not so. Routine acts for most people (dressing, going to work, etc.) are subsidiary parts of a general scheme of life, part of the general conduct of a life which has to maintain itself. It does not seem too much to say that the normal healthy person carries out these routine acts with a certain forward-looking " zest ". Freud gives the following instances, which seem to speak on this point. " A man overburdened with worries and subject to occasional depression assured me that he regularly forgot to wind his watch on those evenings when life appeared too hard and unfriendly. In this omission he symbolically expressed that it was a matter of indifference to him whether he lived to see the next day. Another man, who was personally unknown to me, wrote after a terrible misfortune, when life appeared hard and unsympathetic, that he forgot to wind his watch nearly every day, though previously accustomed to do it almost mechanically. It was only very seldom now that he remembered it, and that was when he had something important and interesting on hand for the next day."[1] Surely we may draw from this the conclusion that for all of us a routine and apparently mechanical act such as watch-winding is ordinarily part of the scheme of life, in which the future is looked forward to with a certain interest. There is too a certain slight but definite pleasure in the mere fact of the recurrence of the expected ; and similarly a slight disappointment and annoyance when the expected order of events is broken. These feelings do exist in this form apart from the specific nature of the expected events. It is probable moreover that the observations reported by Flügel have reference to the feelings that play on the surface of the mental life, and do not

[1] Freud, *Psychopathology of Everyday Life*, 240 (shortened).

pay sufficient regard to moods and sentiments which exist in the background of consciousness over long periods and give a semi-permanent affective colouring to life. One of the observers indeed states that two sorts of mental state, self-feeling and sexual impulse, tend so often to affect consciousness, either acutely for brief periods or for longer periods as a sort of undercurrent, that he was quite unable to do them justice in his record.[1]

We must however in regard to the foregoing make a proviso, of which we shall see the further importance later. While action is directed towards objective ends, that is to say, while it remains in the instinctive stage, there is the possibility, as we have seen, that feeling may remain approximately on the same level of pleasantness throughout. But as action becomes more conscious of its ends, it becomes increasingly possible that value may be thought to reside in the attainment of some more or less distant end. Action will then take rather the form of a movement from a less to a greater value. As we have seen in the case of the will to power, the valuable moment in the end aimed at may, with increasing power of reflection, come to be thought of as a state of the self, of course as determined by its relation to the outside world. To a reflective being moreover, to think of the process of attainment as itself valuable would be, to some extent, to detract from the energy with which the end is sought. The more instinctive conduct is, the more it is directed objectively, pleasure remaining a superadded element. The more reflective and self-conscious conduct becomes, the greater is the possibility that it can appear to the agent as movement from a state of lesser to one of greater value.

Unpleasure follows on the obstruction or frustration of the instinctive impulses; and thus is to be rightly described as always the result of discord or conflict. The impulse still persists in effort towards its end, but is

---

[1] Flügel, op. cit., 352.

met by some obstacle which prevents success or progress towards it. " Mere loss, mere contraction of psychical existence never pains us by itself. It does so only when some element feels itself thwarted and diminished, and for that we must have some positive reaction and tension. If from the world which is dear to me you could isolate one fraction and extirpate it wholly with all its memories and connexions, I should never feel the loss of it."[1] As a rule this state of discord, in which the instinct still persists in fruitless effort to function against an obstacle, is due to some event extraneous to the mind ; for example, the death of a friend thwarting the impulse of love, the competition of others which impedes our attainment of a desired object, the discovery of a fact which conflicts with a hitherto cherished theory. There is fruitless struggle against the knowledge of an unalterable fact. But there are other cases of unpleasure in which the discord must be described as purely intra-mental. If for example a man, either from a sense of public duty or because his friends expect it of him, persists in public appearances on the platform in spite of extreme shyness, he is likely to suffer much unpleasure. What happens is that, in order to attain to an end prescribed by one instinct, he does violence to another, or else, it may be, fear in one form, that of social disapproval, drives him to brave another fear natural to him, that of prominence before a crowd. Here there is conflict between two impulses ; and if one carries the day, the thwarting of the other, as long as it is not wholly obliterated, involves a certain unpleasure.

The mental life of every living being consists, as we have said of its purely sensory side, in an effort to develop and express fully its inborn nature and capacities. It is therefore of the nature of a struggle against the constant tendency to a lower level of activity, towards that dissipation of energy which means a lower level of conscious

[1] Bradley, " Pleasure, Pain, Desire and Volition," *Mind*, Jan. 1888, 5.

life or ultimately its complete extinction. The conflict in the sphere of higher mental activities is not a different one from that in the merely vital sphere. It is the same struggle against the disintegrating tendencies arising from the material with which mind has to deal. The tendency to run down is always present ; every instinctive activity is, as it were, the energizing of a recalcitrant material. Conscious unpleasure occurs when an instinctive impulse, dominant at the moment, is subjected to a thwarting, against which it still persists in an effort to function, but without success in attaining its end. It is possible to consider this state of discord as the intensification of the struggle which always exists, that towards the maintenance of the higher forms of activity, but which in normal circumstances is carried on successfully and without the feeling of opposition.

Fatigue of course occurs in the higher mental as in the sensory sphere. We know little of the physiological condition which underlies a purely mental fatigue, though it is doubtless some state of the central nervous system. When it occurs, continued mental activity becomes difficult. Very often however it is still carried on under the influence of some other impulse, e.g. work may be carried on because of a wish to please others, or because of fear of their censure. As long as such an impulse remains dominant, the activity is continued in spite of the strain and difficulty. The unpleasure which results is perhaps the simplest case of the conflict mentioned above. Sooner or later however the tendency towards cessation of activity is bound to prevail, and the effect in consciousness will be that the mind will turn with aversion from the fatiguing work in which it is engaged. What is sought instead will depend on the nature and extent of the fatigue. In the case of great and general nervous fatigue there is likely to be mere aversion from the present state without any clear idea of what is sought to replace it. Cessation of activity may mean the oncoming of sleep, and in this the mind may acquiesce. But where fatigue is less complete and general, and the higher nervous centres are still capable of functioning to some extent, the tendency, for the time being at least, is likely rather to be towards easier forms of mental activity, involving less concentration and effort ; after a hard day's work, a game, light conversation, easy reading, or mere reverie. All these activities may be described generally as forms of play, that is to say the discharge of the remaining surplus vital energy, taking place in the channels laid down by the bodily and mental constitution, but accompanied by some awareness that the activity is of the nature of a voluntary relaxation and that the whole self is not engaged in the pursuit of any vital end. According to the amount of the surplus energy that is being used up, these forms of activity may be very pleasurable. They will often be thought to be more pleasant than those activities in which the mind engages with its whole force, because in these latter the serious maintenance of life is usually concerned, and thus there is involved a feeling of strain and compulsion, whereas in the easy activities of play there is a feeling of freedom. Yet this pleasantness is itself very largely due to the felt contrast with the fatigue that has preceded in the serious pursuits of life. Most people would, I imagine, have a feeling of descent to a lower level of activity and consciousness, if they gave up their lives entirely to easy pursuits in the relaxed spirit of play, instead of to the working out of the major instincts in their true and more serious form.

It is in connection with this point that we may mention the part played in life by the desire for narcotics, such as alcohol.[1] At all times, for such a highly developed nervous being as man, it is possible that the numerous small stimuli which affect the senses will appear as disturbing and irritating. Especially is this the case when the

---

[1] This subject is introduced chiefly because those writers who, following Freud, make pleasure the result of " reduction of tension " attribute considerable importance in their statements to the pleasure of narcotics. See Bousfield, *Pleasure and Pain*, 67–9.

organism is fatigued after work, presumably because then the nerves, having only a low reserve of surplus energy, are easily exhausted. One of the effects of alcohol is to deaden the irritation derived from these sources. Again in men whose intellect and sensibility are highly developed there is a constant tendency to " worry ", to keep on thinking of the past with regret and the future with anxiety. This also is particularly the case when there is some amount of fatigue and the system does not immediately recover. The mind of the overworked business man continues to occupy itself with the problems of the past day. The effect of the narcotic is in the direction of abolishing these sources of irritation. But at the same time, if taken in moderation, it does not go far enough to cause interference with such an easy activity as social conversation with friends. Such an activity indeed proceeds more easily owing to the removal of the above-mentioned distractions and irritations. Intrusive thoughts, which would arise in relation to others, make us more self-conscious and inhibit the free play of social intercourse, are deadened. We become more simple and direct in our intercourse with others. It is thus that the effect of a narcotic may be to abolish inhibitions and to enable an easy form of mental activity to proceed more directly and simply. The easy form of activity thus forwarded is usually social intercourse, but mere reverie or day-dreaming may be forwarded by the same means. It is in this way that a very large part of the attraction of narcotics is constituted. Often too of course a directly narcotic effect is sought, i.e. the abolition or deadening of unpleasant sensations.

It should hardly be necessary to add that in the sphere of the " higher " feelings, as in those of the sensory order, there is inseparably bound up with pleasure and unpleasure a primary act either of acceptance or rejection. In the pleasant experience that which the mind is striving towards is in course of being attained, so that in such a condition there must always be some energy of self-maintenance. The unpleasant experience is a state of conflict from which the self is endeavouring to pass away in order to restore the condition in which activity is unobstructed. The unpleasant state is therefore essentially one which is rejected.

CHAPTER VIII

THE ÆSTHETIC EXPERIENCE. PLAY

A PRINCIPAL object aimed at in the foregoing has been to show that on the success or non-success of the instinctive conations there follow the feelings of pleasure or unpleasure. But if we are to prove that this is essential to pleasure and unpleasure, we must also start from the other end and show that there are no instances of these feelings which do not fall under this definition. There are a certain number of pleasures, usually held to be of the higher mental order, which might be thought at first sight not to do this. For example it might seem that æsthetic pleasure, depending on the perception of the beautiful in nature or art, is given all at once, and is not dependent on any previous conation. We will therefore now look at the sphere of æsthetics. It is necessary for reasons of space to state our view without discussing the enormous number of varying theories which have been held on this subject.

According to the view taken here the æsthetic experience is not a simple one, but a complex and late-developed form of mental activity, the pleasure which enters into it being the result of a number of factors. In every form of art the first and lowest fact is that given by the sensory material. The material of a picture is made up of colours, that of a piece of music of tones. We have already sufficiently indicated how it is to be believed that the pleasure of single and simple sensations is the result of successful conation, and how it is possible too that some of the pleasures of simple harmonies, i.e collocations of colours or tones, are to be explained in the same way.

Beyond this simple sensory element in æsthetic satisfaction there is to be found a pleasure attached to the element of form. We have already given a partial discussion of this point in treating the instinctive impulse towards knowledge (see pp. 91–2). That form is pleasing which affords a regular scheme easily to be grasped by the mind, in contrast to that which is irregular and pointless, which creates expectations which it does not fulfil. But on the other hand mere regularity and a plain repetition of the previously given appears to us as monotonous, inasmuch as it gives too little exercise for mental activity. The most fully satisfying forms are those in which a variety of elements is synthesized under a governing principle in one unity, so that there is some consciousness of power and ease in transcending and unifying the apparent multiplicity. This is applicable of course not only to spatial patterns, but also to those of tones. There is, I think, no other satisfaction than this attaching to pure form as such.

Through the medium of the apprehension of forms however there are other sorts of pleasure to be created, which are of greater importance. We pass here to the side of art in respect of which it has significance, i.e. represents something other than itself. The distinction is often naturally made between imitative and non-imitative arts, painting, sculpture, and poetry on the one hand, architecture and music on the other. But as we shall soon see, this distinction is not ultimate from the point of view of æsthetics, and there is a way in which the arts, not immediately imitative of nature, yet possess a representative or significant side. We can here refer back to the description given when dealing with the genesis of self-assertive pride. As there stated, the primitive mind tends inevitably to a self-projection into, and a vivification of, external objects. This tendency remains with us throughout life. Immediately and quite unconsciously we tend to project into an object, provided it gives us some sort of initial cue, the same sorts of emotions and feelings which we should have if we were in the position

Q

of that object. There is no awareness that we are reading our own feelings into the object; it appears to us as though it were the object that were infecting us with the feelings. Thus a lofty tower or a mountain peak appears to us as lifting itself and soaring proudly into the sky; Ruskin, I think, spoke of the Matterhorn as tossing itself into the sky like a rearing horse; we have the sympathetic consciousness of power. The torrent is to us angry and impetuous, the slow river lazy and peaceful; and they seem to infect us with those feelings. To take an example from the sphere of human construction, we feel into the column an activity in supporting the beam or other burden it has to carry. The effect is pleasing if it appears to carry it easily and adequately. Any suggestion of top-heaviness, inadequacy, or lack of balance affects us unpleasantly through the same sympathy. There is the same phenomenon even with the simplest forms. A line, if it is irregular and wavers, gives us the impression of weakness, hesitation, uncertainty. An even curve is decided and strong, and may also give us the impression of smooth, easy, and pleasant movement. It is thus for the most part that we get the distinction in pleasurableness between the patterns which we call bold and flowing, and those which are weak and uncertain.[1]

In a great many cases, if not perhaps in all, the suggestion of movement or attitude given us by the object is accompanied by some sympathetic change in the tension of various groups of the voluntary muscles and some sympathetic alteration of breathing and pulse. Adam Smith noted this in his treatment of sympathy. " The mob when they are gazing at a dancer on a slack rope naturally twist and writhe and balance their own bodies as they feel him do, and as they feel that they themselves

---

[1] It is the line itself in which the movement is felt. It is not necessary that there should be any suggestion of the movements, which I, the onlooker, would have to make in drawing the line myself. So experimental observations seem to show. See Valentine, *Experimental Psychology of Beauty,* 46–8.

must do if in his situation."¹ Whether this occurs in all
cases of the sympathetic induction of an emotion is perhaps
doubtful; it is possible that the cognitive element in
these mental states may consist solely in the sympathetic
realization of the situation or imagined situation of the
observed object. But certainly in many cases some actual
incipient movements or attitudes are induced in the
onlooker by the movements which he observes, or thinks
of as occurring, in the external object; and this gives
additional actuality and warmth to the feelings which he
experiences.²

We can now see how in the æsthetic experience it is
possible for impulses which do not in ordinary life obtain
sufficient outlet to obtain some sort of satisfaction. Those
objects are æsthetically pleasing which give an outlet to
impulses which crave exercise. At ordinary times these
impulses remain latent, contributing to the mental life
at most an indefinite restlessness, a vague sense of something wanting. But as we saw in dealing with the sensory
feelings, it is still possible for the moment of satisfaction
to yield pleasure in an acutely conscious degree. Our
instances given above were those of inanimate objects.
But when any art directly represents human forms or
actions, it is of course more obvious that pleasure is
yielded by the satisfaction of subconscious longings and
needs. We enter sympathetically into pictures depicting
figures stately, heroic, tender, etc., into story or poetry
which represents love, adventure, successful ambition;
and so our impulses in these directions, which do not
obtain adequate satisfaction in our ordinary lives, obtain

¹ Adam Smith, *Theory of Moral Sentiments*, chap. i.
² There is an interesting discussion of this point by Groos, *Spiele
der Menschen*, 423–30. It is appropriate, perhaps, to remember
Wordsworth's lines :—

> The floating clouds their state shall lend
> To her; for her the willows bend;
> Nor shall she fail to see
> Even in the motions of the storm
> Grace that shall mould the maiden's form
> By silent sympathy.

it vicariously.[1] We can thus view all these activities as a sort of play.

It may be noted incidentally that in relation to this, the significant side of art, form plays a dual rôle. The composition of a picture, for example, includes two factors. In the first place the form can subserve the meaning in the fact of its lines leading our attention to that part of the picture which in meaning too is most important and interesting. In the second place there are qualities which we feel into the forms and lines, and which they appear to us to possess in themselves. Thus a picture may appear lop-sided if the weight of colour or material is concentrated exclusively to one part. But these qualities ascribed to the forms of the picture may themselves again combine with and subserve the meaning of the work. For example in Piero della Francesca's picture of Christ rising from the Tomb, the lines themselves, merely as a pattern, suggest upward movement. In El Greco's picture of the Agony in Gethsemane, all the lines of the composition are twisted and contorted, so that they reinforce the meaning yielded by the central figure.

The ascription of beauty to the human body takes place, according to our view, because we feel that it represents the balanced and harmonious perfection of our type, and in it therefore our efforts and aspirations towards perfected physical and mental life are fulfilled. It has been described by Lipps as " the free affirmation of life felt in the contemplation of the object ".[2] This is beauty in the narrower sense of the term, and it may be added that, in the fact of the harmony and balance of the perfected type, there is always some possibility of lack of specific character, and therefore of some lack of interest ; a possibility which often comes near to fulfilment in respect of the merely beautiful. That human face or form on the other hand is ugly to me, into the life of which

---

[1] The question of tragedy will come up later.
[2] Lipps, " Aesthetik," in Hinneberg's *Kultur der Gegenwart* (1907), 360.

I feel I cannot enter, which repels as deformed or un-
healthy, or which expresses passions with which I cannot
sympathize.   Here as elsewhere the unpleasure is the
result of a discord.   The perceived body starts in me an
impulse towards the imitation of its attitudes or expressions, and so in the direction of entering sympathetically
into its life.   But this initial impulse is checked by the
fact that it comes into contradiction with the pre-existing
direction and settled character of my mental life.

It is necessary to ask whether this æsthetic sympathy
is different from the ordinary sort of sympathy with persons, which we have already described in dealing with
altruism.   We may in the first place repeat that in all
these cases of æsthetic sympathy there is no conscious
reading by us of movements or feelings into the object.
Æsthetic pleasure would be ruined if we were aware
that we are attributing to the mountain or the spire a
soaring impulse, while in reality it is a dead mass in which
the pressure of all the parts is downwards not upwards.
Coleridge has written some wonderful lines expressing
the general fact that it is we who animate nature, those
in the ode on Dejection which begin :

> O lady, we receive but what we give,
> And in our life alone does nature live.
>
> .   .   .   .   .
>
> We in ourselves rejoice,
>   And thence flows all that charms or ear or sight,
> All melodies the echoes of that voice,
>   All colours a suffusion from that light.[1]

But whatever power we may think he has put into this
statement of the general law, his vindication of man
against nature, as we may call it, it remains true that in
each particular case the occurrence of this thought
would spoil our feeling of the beauty of the external
object.   So far as overt consciousness is concerned, it

---

[1] Intended, I believe, as a direct answer to Wordsworth's views as
expressed in lines such as those quoted above from the poem " Three
Years She Grew ".

seems to us as though the suggestion of feeling or emotion were given directly to us by the object. What is no doubt true is that in the æsthetic experience the distinction between the self and its objects is, while not wholly lost, yet at a minimum. We give ourselves over to the object in æsthetic contemplation and do not distinguish clearly between our own feeling and that which is thought to be suggested by the object. The total situation, for example, when we look at a mountain is one of power and sub-limity. Nevertheless the consciousness of the subject-object relation cannot be entirely lost, and in so far as it exists, it is we who seem to be receiving from the object and not vice versa. It is at this point that we can dis-tinguish æsthetic sympathy from the ordinary sympathy with persons. In everyday life when we sympathize with another there is present the underlying belief in the reality of the feeling or emotion as actually lived by the other ; and so it is experienced as an object which at least tends to demand some reaction of our own, may-be of anger or fear in response to anger, or of tenderness to answer unhappiness, and so on. In the æsthetic experience there is always some detachment from reality in the sense that there is an abandonment for the time being of our will to realize in action the impulses of our own nature. We give ourselves over to the object and live in its life (or what appears to be such), finding that life in agreement or disagreement, as the case may be, with our own impulses, but in any case living out the whole series in an ideal world, not that in which our personal self has to maintain itself against external force and meet the action of other selves with a reaction of its own. Such a detachment from the serious effort of self-maintaining life is given in the work of art by the fact that we are aware from the first of its make-believe character and this realization remains subconsciously with us during our contemplation of it. Of course it is possible to contemplate real persons in the same spirit of æsthetic detachment. But as soon as we begin to treat the anger or suffering or joy of another as real in the sense of requiring a personal reaction of our own, then the æsthetic element in the experience has disappeared. For these reasons it does not seem to me that " Empathy " (as it has been called in translation of the German Einfühlung) is ultimately a different sort of process from sympathy. Some self-projection is the necessary first stage of a fully developed sympathy.

We do not mean to imply by the foregoing that art is nothing but the imitation or restoration in memory of past valuable experiences. The creative artist is one who, possessed by strong impulses which demand some outward expression, finds this expression through the imagination of new objects or situations instead of resting content with those which may occur to him. It is possible for him thus to give others the opportunity of entering into his own valuable experiences, and so of obtaining intenser values than they would be capable of by themselves. And in the mere fact of being given an ideal form, these experiences will differ from those of real life. Every actual experience is subject to checks, limitation, and friction, which spring from its sensory accompaniment and its setting in real life. In ideal construction these drawbacks can to a large extent drop out, and the whole experience can take place in a freer and purer form.

All that is ordinarily called æsthetic experience does not however involve the sympathetic entering into other life. Some forms of such experience are due to more direct suggestion of emotions. The deep blue of the summer sky is pleasing to us partly because it means warmth, open air, absence of constraint, and physical well-being. Hence a similar blue may be pleasing to us wherever seen, because it gives a vague suggestion of these associated ideas. Similarly with any colour that suggests sunlight, or a green which suggests fresh foliage. The beauty attributed to natural scenery is undoubtedly a matter of some complexity, and the whole subject must be considered somewhat uncertain in view of the fact that the æsthetic

judgments of natural scenery are extremely variable.
For instance, to-day we admire some landscapes, such as
mountains and those of a wild and savage character,
by which our ancestors of two hundred years ago were
repelled. No doubt one source of the pleasure given
by natural scenery is this. All civilized people, especially
those who live in towns, but also country dwellers within
their own houses, pass much of their time amid the forms
and colours of man-made objects. In the open country
we feel a certain expansion and freedom as contrasted
with the vague oppression induced when we are surrounded
by walls and buildings. Perhaps it is not fanciful to
believe that our organs of sight have through long ages
become attuned to the forms and colours of natural
objects and do not feel at home with those of artificial
objects. This dissatisfaction with continual perception
of the artificial may be shown in the strong need which
most people have to adorn their rooms with flowers
and plants. Among landscapes there are some which give
more sense of openness and freedom than others, and
which afford a greater variety of natural forms and colours.
These are as a rule considered the more beautiful. At the
same time there are ways in which elements of æsthetic
sympathy enter into the admiration of natural scenery.
Whenever living vegetation is part of the landscape,
there may be some sympathetic appropriation to ourselves of its vigorous and freely developed life. That which
has developed its own life fully and freely can infect us
with a consciousness of fulness of life. Sometimes too
human qualities appear to be suggested by living vegetation. We speak of the rugged strength of the oak, of the
lightness and grace of the birch. We have already dealt
with the sublime, i.e. the sympathetic consciousness of
power, which can be found in natural objects. There is
surely no reason to suppose that the pictured representation of nature by the artist is necessarily capable of being
æsthetically superior to nature itself, i.e. that the artist
can put into his picture more than it is possible for himself

(or another) to see in nature. The æsthetic appreciation of the picture and of nature itself will be fundamentally the same.

A few words must be added on music, as it distinguishes itself from the other arts by handling tones, while they handle visual forms. Music in the first place makes use of sounds which yield sensory pleasure, either intrinsically, or in their relations of harmony to the sounds preceding and following them. With these materials sound patterns are constructed which are capable of yielding the intellectual pleasures peculiar to form perception, e.g. those due to satisfaction of expectations and to the comprehension of details as parts of a single scheme. Beyond this we have the emotional effects of music. It is doubtful if the extraordinary intensity and peculiar character of the emotion which can be produced by music can be adequately explained. It may be due to facts of racial history and inheritance with which we are not fully acquainted. Such explanation as can be offered here is as follows. In the first place the mere repetition of rhythmical sound patterns seems to be capable of arousing a singular excitement, which may possibly be due to coincidence with the rhythms of the bodily life. Beyond this music evokes emotion in two ways. Firstly and principally by the suggestion of movement. Melody and rhythm suggest human gesture movements of all sorts, stately, playful, agitated, and so on. But they can go far beyond this and create ideas of movement which transcend our ordinary experience, swinging, floating, gliding, the rush of a torrent, the soaring of a bird. There is, it seems to me, this fact about the suggestion of movement in music which goes far to explain its peculiar " intoxicating " effect, sometimes soothing and sometimes exciting. By its very nature it suggests movement free from the ordinary impeding factor of some kind of friction, and to some extent that of gravitation also. These limiting factors are left out in the ideas created by music ; the movement suggested is one purified and set free from such ordinary trammels.[1] There is then created in us that feeling which would be capable of accompanying the movement. In the second place the human voice in singing, by the tempo of its utterance and by its timbre, expresses to us the various emotions of the utterer ; and other forms of music, by virtue of their resemblance to the human voice, can suggest to us emotions in the same way, for example, pleading, wailing grief, passionate love, triumphant pride. A concerted piece can give a whole dramatic series of the emotions suggested in all the above-mentioned ways. Doubtless most people in our society live a life in which there is not often given an outlet for the emotions, and at times there will occur in the mind a certain vague dissatisfaction with this ordinary life as dull and flat and a temporary need for something more exciting. Music (like the other arts) takes them temporarily out of their ordinary life by suggesting (in play) the emotions of an exciting and varied life. They live in make-believe for the time a fuller and more varied life, in which outlet is given to all the capacities for emotion. No doubt the emotions mentioned above are not in all cases happy ones, but into the reasons for the value of the tragic we will go later. As the final result of the feelings and emotions aroused in all these different ways, there may be formed a single unified affective state. There is always, it can be maintained, and as we shall see further later, a tendency for the feelings of one class (pleasure or unpleasure) to fuse into a whole in consciousness, producing a result in which the component feelings for the most part disappear. This is the more likely to happen when the different feelings appear as the result of different aspects of one object. What can happen in the case of music is not only such a total state of feeling, but also a unified emotional state coloured in a definite way. The unity of a piece of music must be essentially an affective

[1] Cf. above, pp. 133–4, on the pleasure of frictionless movement. It is for this reason perhaps that the intoxicating effect of music is especially felt in such pieces as Mendelssohn's " Oh for the wings of a dove ", Wagner's " Ride of the Valkyries ", Debussy's " En Bateau ".

unity. Though it may be difficult to specify in detail the means by which it is brought about, yet it does seem that the tones, the form or pattern, and the suggested movement in a musical composition may each severally go to induce the same colouring of emotion, and thus go to build up a unified emotional state of considerable intensity.

It will be appropriate to say something here on the nature of the comic or ludicrous, as it, like æsthetic experience, in its most important aspects, falls under the general heading of " play ". The attitude of play is one in which there is a certain mental relaxation, in which instinctive ends are still pursued, but with a detachment which prevents that pursuit being quite whole-hearted, and so with some consciousness on the part of the agent that he is free, that it is always possible for him to give up the pursuit. We sometimes speak of a pursuit as " not whole-hearted " in the sense that there is distraction by a competing impulse. But this state of mind is not the same as that in play. It is within a total mental situation of the nature of play that the comic arises. Its specific cause is as follows. The initial phase is that of a self-assertion in the " playful " form, when we ourselves set ourselves out in such a spirit to do something big, or when we as onlookers see others prepared to be grand and pretentious, yet do not contemplate them with whole-hearted awe and reverence. The mind is thus prepared in a way for something big and important, with a sense of tension or strain. Then suddenly that which sets out to be great and impressive is turned into something incongruously small and petty, its dignity being thus taken down. There is a sudden relaxation of the mental tension and the surplus energy discharges itself freely in certain otherwise meaningless movements and gestures, those of laughter. This particular form of movement is one for which we cannot fully account. There must be behind it a story of physiological development in the race. It is however obvious that it both serves as a channel for the outlet of the surplus energy, and at the same time itself has a secondary pleasurable effect in stimulating the circulation and general bodily activity. It is the moment of sudden relaxation from strain and release of energy which yields the actual pleasure of the comic. There is always the possibility of a certain moment of disappointment in the comic; and this of course may sometimes be strong enough to prevent the total experience being pleasant. It is quite wrong to find the essence of the comic in the superiority felt when we see the dignity of another suddenly taken down. True humour is laughter *with* others not *at* others. A sense of humour enables us to laugh at our own misfortunes or "takings down", as at those of others. The reason why we do not so often do so is that our own self-assertive pride is for us usually whole-hearted and not playful. It is particularly when we watch the self-assertive pride of another in a make-believe attitude, e.g. at the theatre, and in reading a story, that the initial preparation for the humorous is given. There are some who go through real life in this half-detached and tolerant frame of mind, and it is these who are pre-eminently judged to have a sense of humour. On the other hand those who have devoted themselves with passionate earnestness to the narrow end of some particular reform, are often deficient in the sense of humour, according to the ordinary judgment of men. None of us indeed are inclined to find anything funny in the degradation of that which we regard with deep-seated reverence and affection. I suppose one of the classical instances of the comic is that of the new M.P. who sits down on his own hat after his maiden speech. There is certainly here a taking down of dignity. But the onlookers only find it mirth-provoking because they have been listening to him throughout in an attitude of half-patronizing detachment. It is unlikely that an occurrence of this kind in a debate of intense earnestness, say that on the question of war with Germany, would have provoked much merriment.

There are a number of other activities which fall under the general class of play. Most games are contests between antagonists in some form of strength or skill. In them men endeavour to satisfy the competitive impulse, the will to power, and usually to some extent to have the result confirmed by the applause of others. At the same time games and sports exercise bodily and mental capacities which are inborn in us as the result of racial history, but which in civilized society often obtain insufficient exercise and therefore crave outlet. Such exercise will therefore be pleasant. We only as a rule in any sort of play aim at the end of power or felt superiority over others by a form of exercise which is pleasant in itself, not by one which is monotonous or painful. Outdoor games exercise the body, and in addition give opportunity for practice of various sorts of skill which were in the past of value for self-preservation, and to which probably there is some inherited predisposition, for example accuracy in co-ordinating hand and eye so as to hit a mark with a missile. Indoor games (apart from mere gambling), such as chess and bridge, exercise mental capacities which have been developed as of value in the struggle for existence, for example the power to construct in idea and carry out in practice a detailed plan of action towards an end. To outwit an adversary by a feint or bluff also makes one feel superior to him in mental power. There are also amusements which do not involve a contest against an adversary, such as the solving of puzzles or problems. In these the pleasure is for the most part that of exercise of the mental powers. Puzzles for the most part consist in this, that a series of terms is given with the relations between them, and a missing term has to be found to suit a given place in the series. They thus involve something like a rule of three sum, which requires the capacity for the " eduction of a correlate " or " analogical extension ".[1] There is also to some

[1] See p. 110 above, dealing with the development of the intellectual powers.

extent a consciousness of power yielded by the solution of such problems, inasmuch as the artificially created difficulty presents itself, as it were, in the guise of an obstacle or adversary which is overcome. In these activities, as in the instincts generally, pleasure is found in the process of working out and attainment, not in the end by itself. The mere possession of the end, e.g. the answer to a puzzle, yields no pleasure in itself, but only the fact that by a process, whether long or short, one has worked it out oneself. Otherwise there can be neither exercise of mental capacities nor enhancement of self-feeling. There are forms of bodily and mental exercise which are aimless, not directed to any definite end, a mere random exuberance of bodily movement, or a spinning of trains of ideas in reverie. These forms of exercise may be pleasant as affording some outlet to unemployed energy. But the whole experience is different in character from the exercise which takes place in pursuit of a definite end. The activity is less strenuous, more relaxed, less controlled. Stout has stated that, in the fact of gradual progress towards the result and the exercise of the powers therein involved, is to be found the formal end of an activity, while the result aimed at is the material end.[1] There is a distinction of this kind to be drawn between the factors present in any pursuit. But it seems to me it would be more correct to draw it somewhat differently, i.e. between the pleasure yielded by the consciousness of gradual approach towards a desired end, and the pleasure yielded by the exercise of capacities incidental to the progress. The two are not the same, though in the case of any pursuit each may doubtless contribute to the pleasantness of the total situation. The consciousness of gradual approach is a factor which appertains to the final result ; it is a pleasure of partial attainment. It is possible moreover to seek bodily and mental exercise for its own sake alone, and then it becomes what must be termed a " material " end.

[1] *Manual of Psychology*, 694–5.

PART IV

THE PSYCHOLOGICAL NATURE OF PLEASURE AND UNPLEASURE IN COMPARISON WITH SENSATION

IT will now be our endeavour to define the feelings of pleasure and unpleasure in themselves, as elements of consciousness, and to state their relation to other mental elements. It has long been the custom to divide the psychical facts into the three orders, cognitive, affective, conative. Külpe has suggested in place of this a division into Contents and Functions ; under the former would be included sensations, images, ideas, concepts, everything that is given to the mind and makes up the material of the mental life; under the latter all the modes of reaction to this material, the ways in which we behave to it, attend to it, concern ourselves with it, seek or avoid it, and so on.[1] The former would correspond roughly to what might by others be called the cognitive elements, the latter to the conative. What then is the place of feeling as regards the other two sorts of psychical fact ? Külpe speaks of the feelings rather vaguely as constituting in a certain sense the transition between contents and functions. The point to which our preceding discussion has been directed has been that of showing that the feelings of pleasure and unpleasure are mental elements which arise in dependence on the form in which the mind functions in regard to its contents, i.e. on the form in which it attains (or does not attain) the material ends prescribed by its innate

[1] Külpe, *Vorlesungen über Psychologie*, 128–35.

constitution. If this attempt has been successful, it follows that the relation of pleasure and unpleasure is more directly to the functional or conative side of mental life than to its contents. It is the cognitive elements which primarily constitute the contents which are pursued, maintained, or avoided. But the nature of the feeling, in as far as the difference between pleasure and unpleasure is concerned, does not depend on the nature of these cognitive elements, but on the form of the conative series. Yet it must be admitted that the feeling, even if dependent on, or secondary to, the conation, is not itself identical with it. If we look at those impulses which, arising from the main human instincts, are present in a conscious form in the mind, it can be seen that in these cases, consciousness of a conation as attaining its end is not *identical* with pleasurable feeling. Consciousness of a conation is the consciousness that there is an active direction of the self towards the bringing about of some change, and that this activity is effective or not effective, as the case may be. Consciousness that the self is acting effectively is not the same thing as the feeling of pleasure. In the feeling of pleasure there is added to the knowledge of " effectiveness " a certain peculiar warmth, which we can also term " a sense of value ", but cannot define further ; well as we know it in ordinary experience. The facts are of the same order as those of emotion. Fear is not exhaustively defined as conscious impulse to escape from a given situation, nor anger as the conscious impulse to damage or destroy an object which obstructs us. With both there occurs an element possessing a certain " warmth " or " intimacy " to the self, which we term affective, but cannot further define. Pleasure and unpleasure are then the ways in which the self is affected by the attainment or non-attainment of the ends to which it is innately disposed ; the marks of the peculiar interest and value which it finds in those ends. The same plainly is true of the maintenance of the bodily processes. For the most part these processes are not dependent on our direct co-operation. Intentionally and of set purpose we can as a rule only influence them indirectly, by providing external conditions favourable to them. But, as we have already stated, the conscious self feels itself immediately bound up with their existence and with their normal functioning, in a way which we must take as it appears and cannot further describe or account for. Bodily pleasure and unpleasure are in our view the expression of the interest and value which the successful process of the bodily functions must possess for the conscious self. They are not identical with the acts of primary acceptance and rejection, though such acts always occur with them. They are something additional to the acts, or to any act as such.

In order to defend and substantiate this position, however, it is necessary to consider somewhat more closely the ways in which the feelings differ from and are related to the cognitive contents of mind. For on the view we have stated, it would still appear as though the feelings, though dependent on conation or function, are yet in themselves more of the nature of psychical contents.

In the first place we must subscribe to the opinion of those[1] who have pointed out that feeling is not a quality of sensation, in the sense in which intensity would be described as a quality of all sensation, or in which colour could be described as a quality of visual sensations. These qualities cannot be imagined as abolished without the sensation itself being abolished at the same time. But a sensation taken by itself can be imagined, and indeed does often occur, without a feeling attached to it, even if the total mental state, as we have maintained, always includes some elements of feeling. We may assume then that pleasure and unpleasure are, as component parts of consciousness, separate mental elements, capable of having qualities of their own.

---

[1] See Wohlgemuth, *British Journal of Psychology*, Vol. 8, p. 427.

R

But are they independent mental elements in the same way as sensations are ? Can they exist by themselves apart from cognitive mental elements ? The general opinion probably has been that this is impossible, that, though separable in introspection, they are in fact always secondary or epiphenomenal, arising in dependence on the course of the rest of consciousness, and never without the presence of some cognitive elements. It has, however, also been asserted by others that states of pleasure and unpleasure by themselves do occur. Wohlgemuth writes as follows : " There are also certain states of consciousness, states which we may call ' laissez vivre ', probably identical with the ' dolce far niente ', where introspection, or better retro-introspection, seems to reveal that all we have been conscious of was a state of a merely affective nature, highly pleasant. The cognitive content was, so to speak, nil, or if present, transitory, fleeting, constantly changing and quite independent of the affective content of consciousness, which remained constant." He further gives as instances of the independent existence of affective states, " those emotional dispositions known as moods ", which are apparently able to govern the course of the cognitive contents, suggesting ideas which fit in with themselves, in a cheerful mood, cheerful objects, in a depressed mood, melancholy objects.[1]

In regard to the first statement, that relating to states of " dolce far niente ", it would, I think, probably be agreed that the cases where, as alleged, nothing but an affective consciousness exists are only those of pleasure, not of unpleasure. A generally unpleasant bodily condition must always have some positive sensation, or group of sensations, at its core, something experienced as a disturbance of the normal, from which as it were the general unpleasantness radiates, and from which there is endeavour to escape back to the normal. Indeed, as we

---

[1] Wohlgemuth, op. cit., 428–9.

have already pointed out, a depression of bodily vitality which is general and unresisted does not in itself appear to cause unpleasure. Are there, however, conditions of bodily well-being, resulting in conscious states of pleasure which have no discernible relation to any cognitive content, as in the example given by Wohlgemuth of the " dolce far niente " ? It seems to me that some specific sensations would always be detectable in such a condition of physical repose as that mentioned. The most definite would be those of the gentle tension of the muscles and the slow movement of respiration, as remarked in the quotation from Wundt.[1] In actual individual cases these sensory factors would differ in numberless small ways, and would always owe part of their special character to a felt contrast with previous experiences of stronger tension. It is impossible to consider any state of the bodily sensations as a cut-off whole by itself, without allowing for the fact that it forms a phase in a gradually changing series, the changes being as a rule so gradual as not to be noticed at the time. We should describe ourselves as feeling physically well and happy, both when we recline, in the " dolce far niente " condition, after the midday meal on a warm day in the open air, and also when we are first out of bed on a fresh morning after a good night's sleep. But the experienced bodily state is quite different in the two cases, as we can see by making a comparison by memory. In the second case mentioned there is a diffused state of well-being, doubtless due to rapid circulation, favourable nutritive exchanges, freshness of unexercised sense organs and well-rested muscles. No doubt it is difficult to point to any definitely localized organic sensations. But we can plainly see how such a state is felt to differ from the lazy " afternoon " condition. There is a lightness in the limbs and muscles and a readiness for movement, which contrasts with a heaviness and a tendency towards repose ; also a freshness and alertness of the

[1] Wohlgemuth, loc. cit.

sense organs, principally the eyes, contrasted with a certain sluggishness of the sense organs and a slight "heaviness in the head" in the state of repose. The state of the alimentary canal, it must also be remembered, is a constantly changing one; and there can hardly be any doubt that the phase in which it is makes a difference to the total bodily condition as consciously experienced at any one moment. Even in perfect health and without experiencing any discomfort, it is improbable that anyone feels quite the same before and after a good meal. Meumann, who systematically introspected his own bodily sensations over a period of two weeks, declared that the digestion never proceeded quite without sensation on any day during that period.[1] Sensations from all these various sources go together so as to form a gradually changing mass, which usually constitutes the sensory background to the mental life and makes up the content of what is felt vaguely as a state of physical well-being. It must surely be obvious that the experienced difference between the various states, such as those mentioned, is constituted by sensory or cognitive factors and not by affective factors. If the latter were the case, the states could only differ in degree of pleasantness, and perhaps also in its bodily diffusion. But this could hardly be maintained. What however can be admitted is this, that the relative prominence in consciousness of the sensory and affective factors may vary from time to time. At times the sensory factors may be the more prominent; but also often they may be relatively obscured, though never wholly lost, and there may be present little more than a general feeling that things are going well with one.

The above-mentioned general states of bodily sensation are sometimes described as "moods"; but the word "mood" can perhaps be used here in a somewhat narrower sense. A mood, to follow McDougall,[2] can be defined as the subconscious persistence of an emotion,

---

[1] Quoted by Störring, *Psychologie des menschlichen Gefühlslebens*, 38.
[2] McDougall, *Outline of Psychology*, 359–61.

together with the conation to which it is linked. If an emotion, say anger, has once been excited, there often persists for a time the tendency towards that emotion, though the object which originally excited it has passed away and may have been forgotten. This is particularly the case if the emotion has been at the first moment for some reason or other denied its full expression. In such circumstances we may remain " irritable ", ready to show anger at circumstances which would not ordinarily excite it. It is not easy to see how mere pleasure and unpleasure can persist, at least as the first form of a mood in this sense. The pleasure or unpleasure must have been due in the first place to the satisfaction or non-satisfaction of some definite impulse, e.g. that of self-maintenance in one of its forms, of sexual gratification, or of ambition. As the first form of the mood there will be a persistence or " resonance " of emotion defined in some way, as successful or unsuccessful love or ambition ; and there is likely to be a subconscious persistence also of the cognitive ideas by which the emotion was originally excited. What sometimes does happen however is that in time the cognitive ideas disappear ; and also the affective state itself becomes less specific. A state of disappointed love or ambition may become one of a general mental depression, and any success in a particular pursuit may result in a general mood of happiness. This general affective state may continue for some time as the main factor giving a colouring to the background of consciousness. It is possible that at brief moments such a general state of feeling may become central for attention, but it does not seem possible for this to endure except for a very short time. A mood of general pleasure or unpleasure can also be caused as the result of a sensory feeling after attention has been diverted from the original sensation with its feeling. Störring[1] states that he succeeded in bringing this about by instructing his observers, to whom a pleasant

---

[1] Störring, *Archiv für die gesamte Psychologie*, Vol. 6 (1906), 317–25.

taste had been given, to turn their attention away from the sensation at once. One of his observers reported that all the mental phenomena appeared to be immerged into this state of consciousness (Bewusstseinslage), so that the whole conscious state had through it received a definite colouring. Another that the pleasure is spread over the total content of consciousness, even over the idea of the movement to be carried out.

All these general moods seem to have the power to call up by association ideas akin to them. In a cheerful mood we are said to be liable to think of cheerful things, whether reproductions of past experiences, or phantasy-ideas; and similarly in a depressed mood to think of melancholy things. This is no doubt true, but there is room for question as to the exact form in which these associations occur. It does not seem to me that the mood necessarily plays the same part as a cognitive idea does in suggesting other ideas by association. The psychical order of events can be stated as follows. When we have been made angry and are still in an irritable mood, what-ever events happen to come to us are taken by us in an irritable way, we get annoyed at happenings which would ordinarily not annoy us. In such a mood, if particularly intense, we are further inclined sometimes, in the absence of external stimulus, to go out of our own accord to look for an object on which to exercise anger. The mind, when awake and vigorous, always requires exercise on objects, and in the existing form of its activity it prefers and selects objects suitable to that form. Much the same happens, I think, when the mood is one of mere pleasure or unpleasure. The objects and ideas which come to us, whether through direct external stimulation or by the independent automatic action of association, are coloured by our prevailing mood, appear in that form; and also, it being assumed that there is absence of other stimulus and the mind is still active, requiring objects on which to exercise itself, it will be inclined to look for such objects as are suitable to the mood. It is not of course always the case that we adhere to a mood of depression ; we more often react and look for cheerful objects. Still we do sometimes adhere to melancholy subjects and ideas, feeling that they fit in with the prevalent mental condition, and that it would involve a strain and wrench to turn to the cheerful. It does not seem to me necessary to assume that there underlies all this the activity of a particular brain centre, that for feeling, which, having once been excited in conjunction with other centres, tends thereafter to " drain " towards those centres ; i.e. that we have the occurrence of an association of the automatic or mechanical order, similar to that often taking place between cognitive ideas. A more probable explanation, suiting the facts better, seems to me this. In the first place the original pleasant or unpleasant experience has diffused organic effects of excitation or depression, and these may persist for some time after the original stimulus. This is the case with feelings of higher mental origin, as well as with those of sensory origin. It must account in a large measure for the persistent underlying feeling, which both colours the background of the mental life and seems to give a tone spreading to all other mental happenings. But in the second place there are not only diffused organic effects. The original stimulus is capable of leaving some effects also on the central processes, causing them to run temporarily in either an enlivened and vigorous manner or one that is obstructed and difficult. Such a form, once impressed on the psycho-physical process, can endure with a certain persistence and momentum of its own, and can affect all other processes which occur as the result of external stimulus and associative connections, and as the result of the mind's own need for exercise on objects. There will be a preferential selection of those stimulations (from whatever source arising) which harmonize with that pre-existing form and thus do not disturb its continuance. It is not difficult to think of parallel cases of the influence of forms. If we have heard a certain rhythm in music repeated several times and have become temporarily habituated to it, we are quite likely to believe we find it again in any other series of sounds occurring shortly afterwards, though no sensory factor in the two cases is identical ; and we may also become liable to reproduce it in our spontaneous movements. If the above were to be accepted it would be in conformity with a theory asserting that pleasure and unpleasure are mental elements arising in correlation with the form of the psycho-physical process ; but that, while they do not exist quite separately from the presence of cognitive elements, they are still able to act in some degree of independence of those contents, and exercise an influence on the course of the mental life.

It might be alleged also that an affective state, i.e. a mood, can occur as the result or end term of an associative process, in addition to occurring as the initial term in the way described above. For example, the sight of a place in which I have had many happy experiences may infect me with a general mood of happiness, though I have at the moment no clear memory idea of any of the particular experiences. It is a difficult point to decide in what form, if any, the specific memory ideas are present in such a case as this. I believe in most cases they are present dimly in the background of consciousness. If so, we can have no difficulty in believing that the feeling common to them all can be present in a fused or general form, as the result of such separate ideas, and may be for a short time indeed the most prominent element in consciousness. If it can really be established however that no such memory ideas are present even subconsciously, we should be compelled to formulate an explanation in physiological terms. The nerve centres active in the original experience are, we must believe, re-excited in an incipient way, even if there is no result for consciousness. The incipient excitation of a number of nervous elements in that form which was previously pleasurable might be expected to produce, as a total fused result, a wave of general nervous excitation also in the form which is accompanied by pleasure ; a result which might be intense enough to have results for consciousness. In this however we are touching on the question of affective memory, a matter to which we shall return later.

The question of the result of the direction of the attention to the feelings is, it has usually been considered, one of importance in forming a view of their nature. Undoubtedly if the attention is directed to an ordinary object, a cognitive content, it means that its prominence in consciousness is increased, its intensity, as relative at least to the other contents present in consciousness at the time, is increased. It used to be asserted on the other hand in the discussions of moral philosophy that the attempt to concentrate attention on the pleasure element of experience is self-defeating ; that the pleasure disappears if we try to think of it exclusively without also attending to the objective side of the experience. In such discussions this was called the " Paradox of Hedonism ". An attempt at more accurate psychological observation led to the following result being formulated by Zoneff and Meumann.[1] If by attention it is only meant that the subject tries to bring the feeling as far as possible into consciousness, if there is, as it were, a surrender to it (Hingebung), then the feeling, pleasure or unpleasure, is intensified. If on the other hand it is meant by attention that the subject tries to make the feeling the object of a psychological analysis, reflecting for example whether the feeling is more pleasant or not, then the feeling is decidedly weakened, if not altogether destroyed. As regards the main point this result seems to be supported by later experimental observations. One of Wohlgemuth's observers states that by attention in the first place he simply means to make prominent in consciousness. By attending to a feeling in this way he did intensify it. But he failed in his attempts to adopt a critical and analytical attitude towards the feeling, i.e.

---

[1] *Philosophische Studien,* Vol. 18 (1903), 73.

in trying to split up the feeling into its component parts and discover its real nature. In such cases he found himself attending to some cognitive constituent of the experience.[1] Another observer states that by attending to an object he means to bring it before consciousness in such a way that it is the predominant element in the experience. In adopting this attitude in regard to a feeling it became as a rule more intense. He failed however in attempts to direct the attention on the feeling element to the complete exclusion of everything else ; there were always cognitive elements present as well. On the other hand in the attempts to concentrate attention exclusively on the cognitive elements there was often very little feeling present.[2] Wohlgemuth's own conclusion is that, if a feeling element is attended to as belonging to a cognitive content or as part of a situation or complex, it is intensified and becomes clearer ; but if an attempt is made to focus the attention upon it to the exclusion of its cognitive concomitant, the feeling is destroyed.[3] Spearman, as the result of some experimental observations, concluded that although pleasure and unpleasure usually occur in a manner fairly describable as " subjective ", nevertheless many persons —with sufficient training perhaps nearly all—are able to render even these affective states objective at the very instant of their occurrence.[4] In all this, so it would seem, in spite of minor differences, there appears to be agreement that feeling differs from a cognitive content in respect of its relation to attention ; and it would seem that the difference lies in just those points where it would be expected, if the feeling were essentially subjective, a self-state. To direct exclusive attention to a cognized object, or to endeavour to compare it with other objects and analyse its constituents, is *not* to diminish its prominence

[1] Wohlgemuth, *Pleasure—Unpleasure*, 66–8 and 222–4.
[2] Wohlgemuth, op. cit., 133–4 and 222–4.
[3] Op. cit., 224.
[4] Spearman, *Nature of Intelligence and Principles of Cognition*, 236. As to the exact meaning of this objectivation, we add some remarks below.

in consciousness or detract from its apparent intensity, but just the contrary. On the other hand to endeavour to direct exclusive attention to a self-state would be to destroy it, inasmuch as it is only called out by and fed by an objective situation. In the critical and analytical attitude too there is involved an attempted attitude of the self in relation to the feeling ; and we should not expect it to be possible that this attitude should be able to exist simultaneously with the self-state involved in the feeling. The whole case is closely parallel to what happens in emotions such as fear and anger. If we tried to make our own anger condition the object of our thoughts, and ceased to think of the objective cause that had aroused it, our anger would tend to disappear ; as it would too if we tried to analyse and criticize the angry emotion. The only way in which these states of feeling and emotion can be intensified is by a sort of intentional giving oneself up to the total situation, including the object and the affective accompaniment ; though even this is only possible for a short period. Anger will tend to disappear unless sustained by the thought of its original object.

The arguments used above may be thought to be affected by the question of the co-existence of feelings, inasmuch as it might be urged that two attitudes of the self would exclude each other. Wohlgemuth, as the result of a large number of experiments, carried out of course with feelings of sensory origin, concluded that two or more feeling elements, whether like or unlike, can co-exist in consciousness.[1] On the question of fact we might point out that there are some investigators who dispute Wohlgemuth's results in this matter and hold that at present there is no acceptable evidence that affective processes co-exist.[2] We will not go here into this question of the correctness of the observations. We can accept

[1] Wohlgemuth, op. cit., 185-90.

[2] See P. T. Young's articles, *American Journal of Psychology*, Vol. 29 (1918), 237-71 and 420-30 ; *British Journal of Psychology*, April 1925, 356-62, and Wohlgemuth's reply, same journal, Oct. 1925, 116-22.

Wohlgemuth's observations as correct, and still hold that they do not tell against the view that even in sensory pleasure and unpleasure there is involved an attitude of the self, that which we have described as the " moment " of warmth and value, together with a primary acceptance or rejection.

It seems to me quite possible to have two sensations simultaneously and be aware at the same time that we are liking or disliking each separately. It also seems to me possible, though likely to be less frequent, that a pleasant sensation and an unpleasant one should co-exist; and that we should be aware at the same time of a liking for the one and a dislike for the other. Ordinary opinion would certainly be in favour of this, e.g. that we could experience at the same time a sweet taste in the mouth which pleased us, and an ache in the finger which displeased us. The point really seems to depend on the strength of the conative tendencies involved; and it is our opinion that the primary acceptance and rejection of which we speak have not necessarily that strength as conative tendencies which would mean the complete invasion and occupation of the conscious self. Some confirmation of this line of argument may be found in one of Wohlgemuth's results, to the effect that it seems easier for two pleasures to co-exist than two unpleasures; for as he states, in agreement with ordinary opinion, the conative tendencies in unpleasure are much stronger than those in pleasure.[1] According as a conation of any strength is involved in the primary attitude, and especially if the emotions of fear or anger develop from it, then it is plain that this will tend to occupy consciousness completely and to exclude other mental elements. We find a number of reports by Wohlgemuth's observers which exemplify this. In particular the unpleasure aroused by pain sensations or by smells, usually accompanied by strong conative tendencies, is on many occasions

---

[1] *Pleasure—Unpleasure*, 190 and 240.

reported as swamping either the feeling tone of another sensation occurring at the same time or the sensation itself as well. An example that may be quoted is Experiment Y. 141 (simultaneous Galton whistle and pinch with forceps on back of hand). " Both sensations were unpleasant, the pinch sensation the more so. The pain sensation quickly arose with the pinch and was very unpleasant ; strong impulse to withdraw the hand. I had a strong desire to look at my hand, which was inhibited. The pain sensation occupied nearly the whole of consciousness. I was only vaguely aware of the auditory sensation and sometimes this seemed to disappear altogether. It was only by attending hard to the auditory sensation that I could get both sensations in the focus of consciousness. When not attending directly to the auditory sensation it seemed to have no feeling tone, and when directly attended to the feeling was not clearly marked off from that of the pain sensation. I found it very difficult to direct the attention voluntarily to the auditory stimulus, the pain sensation was so predominant."[1] There are also, it is true, certain reports in which it appears to be stated that a conative tendency due to an unpleasant sensation co-existed with the feeling tone of another sensation.[2] And there are others in which it is stated that the feeling tone of an emotion, due to the stimulus or the general situation, co-existed with, and was distinct from, the feeling tone of the sensation itself.[3] It can be admitted that a phenomenon of this kind is not impossible; but it is plain that it is somewhat abnormal. This is plainly shown in the report No. Y. 149. In this the observer states that when a pleasant tactual sensation occurred simultaneously with an unpleasant pain sensation, which latter was accompanied by a strong impulse

---

[1] Other examples are W. 88, 98, 113, X. 76, 107, 123, Y. 112, 126, 143, Z. 145, 153, 154, 155, 161, 165. There is one instance of a pleasant sensation having a similar monopolizing effect, X. 144. This seems uncommon, but possible.

[2] W. 106, 107, Y. 146, 149.

[3] W. 76, 115, Z. 179.

to withdraw, the latter swamped the former, and the feeling tone of the tactual sensation could only be made to reappear simultaneously by a special concentration of attention on it. This however was an act carried out under the motive of the instructions given, to which it would probably be difficult to find a parallel in ordinary life.

As stated above, Spearman reached the conclusion that many persons are able to render affective states objective at the moment of their occurrence, and that training improved this capacity. In Wohlgemuth's conclusions about co-existence of feelings we seem to find something similar. Of his four observers, two failed to experience feelings as co-existent in the first experiments; and as the experiments continued began to find co-existence with some frequency.[1] It seems likely, though Wohlgemuth does not draw this inference, that the possibility of experiencing two or more feelings as co-existent depends in the main on the attitude of the observer, i.e. on whether he is able in some sort to " objectify " the feeling elements. The observers often state that feelings are localized in the body, more especially those arising with the cutaneous sensations and with taste and smell, rather than those with sight and hearing. Wohlgemuth concludes that this localization is dependent on the attitude of the observer towards the feeling element; the more his attitude allows him to objectify the feeling element, the easier it is to localize it (though it is possible the relation may be the reverse, objectivation depending on localization.)[2] In regard to all this it seems to me that the necessary conditions of these laboratory experiments must often make it extremely difficult to obtain normal results on such subjects as feeling and emotion. The natural course of the experience of sensory pleasure or unpleasure is this : they arise as the accompaniment of a certain stage in the process by which the conation of a particular sense organ, or other nervous tract, becomes the attitude

---

[1] Op. cit., 185–90.   [2] Ibid., 207.

and conation of the conscious self. But the experience still appears as having its origin and focus in the given nervous tract, though no doubt to a greater degree with some forms of sensation than others, e.g. with cutaneous more than with visual or auditory sensations. There can surely be no doubt that in these experiments the effect of the instructions given, together with the general frame of mind caused in one about to introspect in a psychological laboratory, would be to induce a spectacular and detached attitude in the observer. The development of the feeling process is likely to be arrested before the rise of the full emotional and conational phenomena which would otherwise occur. The observer might find himself able to introspect and observe the feeling as a quasi-isolated and local phenomenon, before it has progressed so far as to involve an attitude of the whole conscious self. One of Wohlgemuth's observers seems to me to express this on one occasion when he states, in regard to sour and bitter tastes given simultaneously, " Curious feeling of pleasure accompanied the experience from the reflection that I was enduring these unpleasant experiences so dispassionately and disinterestedly, as if they were not my experiences ".[1] From the mode of expression we seem to be justified in inferring that the attitude, though not the reflection thereon, was present throughout this observer's experiments. We also find a number of instances in which observer W. mentions a " spectacular " or " passive " attitude. (Examples are Experiments Nos. 4, 8, 28, 39, 42, 52, 59, 76, 101, 110, 126, 127, 130, 131.) But we need not infer that, in those instances where it is not mentioned, the attitude was totally absent. It seems legitimate to believe that the influence of the instructions and the laboratory atmosphere must have continuously affected the observer's general attitude of mind to a greater or less extent. This attitude of mind is not likely to occur in exactly the same form in ordinary life. Something

---

[1] Wohlgemuth, op. cit., 84, Expt. X. 86.

however rather closely parallel to it does occur. We have noted above[1] that it is possible in ordinary experience for sensory unpleasure to occur in an incomplete form, because another dominant affective attitude is already in existence. In the cases with which we are now concerned the dominant attitude preventing the complete development of feeling would be that of the psychological observer. There may also take place what P. T. Young has called the " meaning-error ". He considers that some of his observers reported pleasure when in truth there was only an inference of pleasant feeling from the awareness of an object that has been pleasant or that usually is pleasant, i.e. an object that carries the meaning of pleasure. Some of his observers actually expressed this distinction. " You assume, I suppose, that honey is pleasant, but I don't think it is in this situation." " There was a sensation of warmth with anticipation that it might become unpleasant, and there was a pressure that I recognized as an experience that was supposed to be unpleasant, but the experience was neither agreeable nor disagreeable."[2] In ordinary life too we may sometimes describe an object as pleasant or unpleasant, when in truth we are only going on the basis of past experience, and a noticeable feeling at the actual moment may not be present.

We remarked above, when discussing the effects of music,[3] that there is a constant tendency for similar feelings, arising simultaneously but in connection with different sensations, to fuse into one whole, resulting in one attitude of the self. This tendency is often reported by Wohlgemuth's observers.[4] It may occur when neither feeling, with the conative tendencies involved, is of sufficient intensity to monopolize consciousness. It is especially likely to occur when both feelings are connected with

[1] See p. 66.
[2] P. T. Young, *American Journal of Psychology*, Vol. 29 (1918), 261.
[3] See pp. 234–5.
[4] Op. cit., 197–8.

sensations referable to one external object. But this does not seem to be an essential condition, for in Wohlgemuth's observations numerous examples of fusion are given with feelings arising from different objects. That fusion is reported in these observations less frequently than co-existence must be ascribed to the already mentioned conditions of such experiments. In ordinary life examples of the fusion of similar feelings seem often to occur. To one lying in the open air on a fine summer afternoon there may come a number of sensory stimuli, each of which is pleasant in effect, the warmth of the air, the colours of sky, foliage, and flowers, the song of the birds, and with these a general sensation of bodily well-being. The feelings resulting from all these sensations will probably as a rule blend into a total state of contentment, in which we do not distinguish different components. An often-quoted example of this blending of feelings is that which results from the bodily sensations, the Gemeingefühl, as it is called by Wundt and Lehmann.[1] A number of different sensations from the body may have their effect on this. But it is almost invariably the case that there is a fusion into a total feeling of bodily well- or ill-being, in which the various feeling components of the blend are hardly to be distinguished. In the resultant there is also to some extent a summation as well as a blending. The total feeling is within certain limits more intense by reason of the addition of the partial feelings, though of course any accurate calculation in this respect is out of the question. In this tendency towards a blending we cannot, it is true, find a criterion which distinguishes feeling definitely from sensation. For it is a characteristic of some sorts of sensation, particularly those less easily localizable in space, i.e. sound and smell, that when simultaneous, they blend into wholes in which the components are often not easily separated out. Nevertheless it can be maintained that a tendency towards a unitary state is a

---

[1] Lehmann, *Die Hauptgesetze des menschlichen Gefühlslebens*, 265–6.

S

characteristic which we should expect to find if the feelings are dependent on the form of the reaction by the self, even if such a characteristic may be also shared by certain sensations.

The general opinion would probably be that opposite feelings, i.e. pleasure and unpleasure, do not fuse into a total resultant which is a " mixed " feeling, though they may alternate very rapidly in consciousness. Wohlgemuth relies on seven statements by his observers to prove that there can be a fusion of opposites into a mixed feeling.[1] If we look at the actual statements, we see that in four of the seven the observer states that there was a total state, predominantly pleasant or unpleasant ; and that in another the experience is described as " very baffling ". These few statements, in themselves so far as I can judge far from definite, hardly seem sufficient to prove the point that opposite feelings really fuse, if one has in view the large number of the experiments that were made with simultaneous stimuli, opposite in feeling tone. In ordinary life we often say that we are uncertain whether we like an object or not. Lehmann gives as an example a scheme of decoration, in which we find the colours pleasing and the arrangement or form unpleasing.[2] In such a case our hesitation in deciding means that we oscillate rapidly between the two alternatives. At one moment, if we are attending more to the colours, the effect is pleasant, at another, when we are attending to the form, it is unpleasant, though the unattended-to aspect remains in the background of consciousness. It is the same as when we hesitate between two contradictory opinions. The two do not form a single " mixed " opinion, but compete in consciousness. Another similar example is that given by Störring, a work of art which is pleasing on the whole, but in which we seem to find some one defect.[3] In looking at such a work of art our state of mind

[1] Wohlgemuth, op. cit., 199–200.
[2] Lehmann, op. cit., 268.
[3] Störring, *Psychologie des menschlichen Gefühlslebens*, 117–18.

on the whole is likely to be one of pleasure, but the un-pleasing element is likely to remain as a constant factor in the background of consciousness, even when not specially attended to, detracting from our enjoyment of the whole. It would surely be unreasonable to speak here of " fusion ". The relation is rather one of sub-traction, in which the elements of positive and negative value are related as plus and minus. A supposed blending of pleasure and unpleasure conveys to me a very indefinite idea ; and so far as my own introspection is concerned, it does not seem to correspond to anything which I actually experience. We shall find it necessary to recur to this question later in discussing the question of varieties of feeling other than pleasure and unpleasure. At present however we may feel justified in concluding that there is a strong tendency for simultaneous feelings of one sort, either pleasure or unpleasure, to sum themselves and blend into a total feeling ; while simultaneous feelings of different sort, pleasure and unpleasure, act rather as contradictories, each preventing the rise of the other. In both respects the view of the feelings as modes of affection of the reacting self seems to be confirmed.

A further point, in regard to which the difference be-tween cognition and feeling has been discussed, is the question whether there are memory-images of feelings in the same sense as that in which there are memories of cognitive contents. The general opinion among psy-chologists has undoubtedly been that there are no such memory-images of feelings, and that the feeling arising with an image or idea is always a present feeling, not to be distinguished by any inner criteria from that which arises in dependence on the present cognized situation. Ribot, admitting that most psychologists hold this view, concluded for himself that while the emotional memory is nil for the majority of people, some are capable of a true memory of feelings and emotions.[1]   Lehmann[2] and

---

[1] Ribot, *Psychology of the Emotions*, 160, 171.
[2] Lehmann, *Die Hauptgesetze des menschlichen Gefühlslebens*, 221.

Wohlgemuth[1] both hold that no memory-images of feelings can be shown to exist. The matter can be stated as follows, I think, in accordance with the general view of the nature of feeling taken herein. Let us assume that what is recalled is a total past situation, which on its first occurrence included both cognitive elements and those of conational and affective character. In such a recall the sensory images are known as such solely by reason of the fact that they contrast with a present reality. The difference of the image from the present impression consists according to Stout in several factors : (1) it is not continuous with and bound up with the actual sensibility of the moment, (2) it has a lower degree of impressional intensity, (3) it is relatively indistinct and schematic, (4) it is fluctuating and does not compel attention by its persistence, (5) it does not vary with our present motor adjustments.[2] Of these, impressional intensity and persistence may not unreasonably be considered the essential differences from which the others spring. The question then naturally arises whether it may not be possible to have a memory-idea of a past situation in which both the cognitive elements and the conational and affective elements contrast by their relatively lesser intensity and persistence with the elements of the present situation, i.e. in which the strivings and feelings share with the sensory elements in the general character of unreality as images. Theoretically this does not seem to be impossible, if it is possible for the different feelings arising in connection with two present sensations to be present in consciousness simultaneously under the conditions already stated. No doubt the differences between the present cognitive percept and the image are more striking. There can be no difference between feelings corresponding to that of distinctness between percept and image. But it does seem as though in fact we can look back on a past situation with some memory of the emotions which then

---

1 Wohlgemuth, *Pleasure—Unpleasure*, 218–20.
2 Stout, *Manual of Psychology*, Book IV, chap. 1.

moved us, and realize at the same time that they are now
past and only recur in a pale and shadowy form as contrasted with the vivid hopes and fears which compose
the centre of our present conscious life.   Ribot quotes as
an instance of affective memory a statement by Sully-
Prudhomme, that when he remembered the emotions
aroused in him by the entry of the Germans into Paris in
1871, he found it impossible not to experience the same
emotions afresh.[1] This however is plainly a case of a present emotion or of the persistence of the same emotion over
a long period.   The true memory of an emotion may have
existed in a Frenchman, able in 1919 to remember 1871,
and to contrast the old feelings as past and unreal with
the vivid reality of the present ones.   It would be somewhat arbitrary to assert that all we ever remember in
such cases is the cognitive fact that we expressed our
feelings, i.e. that we image ourselves as expressing the
feeling by gesture or word, and so infer the past feeling.
Introspection in these cases seems a difficult matter and
its results perhaps somewhat uncertain.   But it seems to
me that it is difficult to assert that we have in regard to
memory-images a definite difference between cognitive
contents and feelings.   The matter too has some bearing
on the general question of the nature of desire and aversion and we shall have to recur to it in that connection.
We shall then, I think, see further reason to believe that
together with the cognitive memory-images of the past
there may recur traces of the previous feelings and conations, which contrast as slight and ineffectual with the
feelings and conations relating to present sensory fact.

    We shall be justified, it may be hoped, in concluding
that pleasure and unpleasure, at least in their complete
form, are subjective mental facts, states or determinations of the self.   Probably no one would deny this of the
feelings which arise in connection with the main conscious
human instincts.   But we can agree that feelings of

---

[1] Ribot, op. cit., 154.

sensory origin are in many cases treated as having a local origin and centre, that there is an incomplete or arrested form in which they are localized, and that in that form they can also with some practice be objectified at the moment of their occurrence. The view that pleasure and unpleasure are subjective states used indeed generally to be considered as one borne out by immediate introspection. For Lotze, apart from pleasure and pain, our knowledge of the difference between the self and its objects would not be distinguishable from that of the difference between two objects; we should not have attained to self-consciousness in the form we know it. Our own self would only be one amongst objects of equal value; " the intimacy, with which in our actual self-consciousness we feel the infinite worth of this return upon ourselves, would still remain unknown and unintelligible." It is pleasure and pain which yield the vividness and force with which this image (that of the self) is felt as different from all else.[1] Wundt too states that, while we objectify sensations, we at once and directly grasp the feelings as what they are, our own subjective experiences, which at the same time mean the way in which we react to the objective impressions given in the sensation.[2] The ordinary opinion and language of men would undoubtedly support the view that we are immediately conscious of pleasure and unpleasure as affections or determinations of the self. While the feelings thus may be regarded as self-states, correlated with a certain form of the psycho-physical process, it is also plain that by an act of abstraction, as a rule taking place in retrospect, they can be distinguished as separate mental elements from the total conscious state in which they occur. In the mere fact of a separate name having been given to these feelings there must have been the work of human minds able in some degree to effect that abstraction. They were able to look back at

---

[1] Lotze, *Microcosmus*, I, 250; cf. II, 680 (translated Hamilton and Jones).

[2] Wundt, *Physiologische Psychologie* (6th ed.), II, 366; cf. I, 411.

that peculiar element of "warmth" and "value", which constitutes the feelings of pleasure and unpleasure, in some abstraction from the sensations and conations with which it was necessarily connected. Animal minds, incapable of speech and always immersed in the course of their instinctive impulses, could never be capable of any trace of such ideas. Moreover, while every mental state includes both cognitive and affective elements, it is possible for the relative prominence of these in consciousness to vary. There are times, as we have seen, when the feelings can be the more prominent and the cognitive elements relatively in the background, though this can be only for short periods. This can be so with any emotion. When there is something of the nature of an intentional self-surrender to an emotion such as anger or grief, the fact of anger or grief may be for brief periods the main fact for consciousness, the external fact or situation to which the emotion is related being for the time less prominent. It is also possible, as we have seen, that the pre-existing conation on which the feeling is dependent, may have been latent and subconscious, and thus that the feeling may appear *ex abrupto* as apparently an independent fact of consciousness. This can occur not only in connection with sensation, but also in regard to some of the major instincts, such as sexual love. In these various ways then pleasure and unpleasure become elevated from their dependent status, and come to be conceived as independent and substantival facts of consciousness.

PART V

PLEASURE AND DESIRE. OTHER CO-ROLLARIES. IDEO-MOTOR ACTION. THE RELATIVITY OF FEELINGS

WE may now ask how the conclusions arrived at affect the question of the nature of desire, that is to say whether in any sense pleasure and unpleasure are the ends or the motives of action. Let us remark in the first place that pleasure and unpleasure can accompany ideas without any tendency to action arising. A memory of the past may be nothing more than a pleasant dream. It may as such be highly pleasant. Alfred de Musset indeed, in his poem " Souvenir ", asserted that pleasure of memory is something more real than that of present experience :

> Un souvenir heureux est peut-être sur terre
> Plus vrai que le bonheur.

He meant no doubt that, immersed in the present experience, we are often less able to realize happiness than when we look back on it afterwards. Be this as it may, the pleasant dream is something that we dwell on for itself and which does not move to action directed towards a present change. Similarly with the memories of unpleasant experiences. There must no doubt go with these some reinstatement of the previous conative elements, the attitude, that is to say, of dislike and rejection. But in so far as the ideas are recognized as pure memory-ideas, not having an immediate relation to present facts with the more urgent and vivid conations connected therewith, the conative elements will only be reinstated in a faint and inchoate form, which will not influence present action.

Actual desire can, in our view, spring only from some existent craving or other form of conation. The fact that a pleasant sensory fact occurs means, as we saw,[1] that a craving, which pre-existed in a slight form, is awakened into consciousness and is satisfied either rapidly or slowly while the sensation lasts. After a few experiences of this kind, say of eating a sweet, the various elements of the experience, the visual, olfactory, and gustatory sensations, which occur simultaneously or in close connection, will by the ordinary laws of association tend to coalesce into a whole; and if one of them occurs separately it will be likely to suggest the others. Suppose then that, as frequently happens, the visual and olfactory sensations of the sweet occur again by themselves, while the nervous elements of taste are already in that slight and subconscious state of tension and craving which we have described. The result will be a suggestion of the craving which was experienced as satisfied on the previous occasion, and this will, as it were, come to meet the present slight craving and will intensify it, at least relatively to the other conscious elements present at the time, so that it becomes fully conscious. When this craving is combined with a more or less definite idea of the end to be attained, we speak of it as desire. Of course if the taste nerves are not already prepared by a condition of tension and craving, i.e. if they have recently been satiated, the suggestion of the craving given by the visual or olfactory sensations will remain slight and of no effect. In such circumstances, with human beings capable of " free " ideas, it is possible that gustatory images may arise without conscious desire. With animals, so far as we know, this would not be possible; the object which does not provoke craving remains probably uninteresting and little noticed. It is in fact the existence of the subconscious craving which determines whether for human beings the suggestion of a pleasant experience turns into an active desire or remains only a passively entertained idea.

[1] See pp. 16–18.

An analysis on the same lines may be applied to more complex instances of human desire. A man, let us say, engaged in office work in the city reads a book or sees a picture which reminds him of holidays spent by the sea or among the mountains. Suppose that at the time he is happy in his work, keenly interested in what he is doing, and not unduly fatigued, the idea of the holiday is likely to remain just a subject of passive reverie, and there is no reason why it should not be entertained as pleasant in momentary alternation with, or interruption of, the interest felt in his work. But a different state of affairs may exist. It is possible that there may be stirring in him certain needs and strivings of which he is not yet fully conscious. He may be feeling a vague, half-conscious dislike of the confined visual outlook of the town, with its sense of oppression or of being shut in ; his muscles may be craving for exercise ; and his work, even if not yet actually fatiguing, may be giving some hint, in lessened zest, of unpleasure to come. In these circumstances the idea of the holiday, if it is suggested, will be that of an experience which, when it occurred, satisfied in the course of its progress those very needs of which up till now he has only been obscurely conscious. The idea of the holiday includes the idea of the needs, inasmuch as they came into it as progressively satisfied. Hence it is likely to suggest anew and to intensify those cravings which actually pre-exist ; and these will possess all the insistence and force derived from present sensory fact over against the idea of the needs as satisfied, which will possess only the relatively pale and unsubstantial form of existence connected with the memory-image. It is thus that what we call conscious desire for the holiday arises. We may thus see, not only that desire for pleasure is not an original principle of action, but also that it is not in truth the pleasure which acts so as to confirm or " stamp in " the tendency to perform an action again. No doubt it often seems as though the memory of an action which was very pleasant attracts to the repetition of it in proportion to the amount of the pleasure. Partly this is due to the idea of the value of pleasure, to which we shall come shortly. Apart from this the attraction of the pleasant idea must be due to the following facts. The fact of a high degree of pleasure having been experienced previously meant that in the experience there was then a very intense discharge of mental energy. When the memory of this experience recurs, it includes within itself a reinstatement of the tendency to discharge of energy in the same direction and with corresponding force. This tendency will be the more likely to be effective in awakening from a latent condition such cravings as already exist. If there is a memory of a past experience as only slightly pleasant, it means that the impulses then given outlet and exercise were lacking in strength, and their reinstatement now will be less likely to vivify a present craving. We are of course only speaking of cases in which there is memory of some happening as pleasant. The mere clearness of a memory-image has no effect in causing a desire for the reinstatement. On the contrary the more clearly the idea of a possible experience is present, the less is likely to be the desire for the actual experience. Vividness of representation by itself detracts from the keenness of desire.

Ideas of unpleasant experience affect present action in a less complex way than that described above for pleasure. Any unpleasant experience at the time of its occurrence includes within itself at least a primary act of rejection with aversion. If it is revived in idea, the dislike or aversion will recur also, but as long as the ideas are regarded purely as such and as having no direct relation to present fact, only in an inchoate and ineffectual form. Sometimes however, if the experience was of an extremely unpleasant character, the conation will take the form of an aversion from entertaining the idea ; and there will be a tendency to exclude it from consciousness and forget it. An idea of such an experience may have two kinds of relation to present fact. In the first place the present situation may appear as one threatening to lead to the actual recurrence of the unpleasant experience. In that case aversion and a conation of avoidance will be actively reinstated. In the second place the unpleasant experience may be regarded as definitely over and as contrasting with the present situation, in which it has been got rid of. In that event it may be possible to dwell on it in idea with something like satisfaction, arising from the fact that the conation of avoidance has been successful.

When intellect has reached a somewhat advanced stage the feeling element, as we have pointed out, can be regarded in abstraction from the total mental state in which it occurs; and it may also be temporarily the most prominent fact in consciousness. It would be therefore possible in any case of desire, where there is a clear idea of the end sought, that the pleasure should be envisaged as a part at least in the end, just as it is possible to guide any pursuit by what is rather a mark or sign of the object aimed at, than the object itself. The idea that men in their actions aim at pleasure as an end is also apparently confirmed by what is in effect an act of further reflection. To one looking back on any experience it appears that the feeling-element of pleasure is that which has given it value. Without the warmth of conscious pleasure the experience is conceivable as a cold mechanical affair, a mere awareness of the effective attainment of what was prefigured in the purposing mind. We shall have to recur to the question of value shortly. But it appears difficult to deny that in fact it is the glow of pleasure in which consists for conscious beings the value of the experiences of success or effectiveness. Without going so far as to think the matter out to its philosophical justification, yet people do ordinarily in something like this way come to think of pleasure as an end which can be pursued for its own sake. Thus we speak of others as " living a life devoted to pleasure "; or a person may say of himself: " I want to be happy, to enjoy myself, to have a good time ". The sort of life indicated in such expressions is in fact something like the following. We speak of a person living for pleasure who is inclined always to satisfy the strongest instinctive impulse of the moment, and so act in the line, as it were, of least resistance. The description appears as plausible, because, in satisfying the impulse uppermost for the time being, the agent is also in fact acting in the direction of the greatest amount of momentary pleasure; and the pleasure will appear as that which gives value to such a life. If on the other hand a man devotes himself whole-heartedly to the end of success in some one pursuit (even if it be only some particular form of sport), we should not be inclined to speak of him as living for pleasure, because often for the sake of his main end sacrifices would have to be made of other instinctive ends also valuable in themselves, and thus temporary unpleasure may be incurred. In a highly organized society it is as a rule possible for a certain number of persons, relieved of the necessity of working for their own support, to find occupation in giving an easy form of satisfaction to the impulses which are strongest for the time being, guarding themselves at the same time by a certain moderation from the discomfort involved in any serious conflict with law or public opinion. A life of this sort in our own time would be occupied for the most part with various sports and games, some attention to art and literature, and light social intercourse, together with the satisfactions of the bodily appetites, food and sex. In these ways some exercise is given to most of the innate capacities of man. For sports and games, as we have seen, afford an outlet for a number of the instinctive needs, while social intercourse may be considered as an easy way of satisfying the gregarious instinct, without involving any intense absorption in the interests of others, or any need of real sacrifice for their sake. The sexual desire, which comes into a life of this sort, will naturally appear as having pleasure for its end; as the tendency will be to make it terminate with the sexual act itself with its high degree of sensory pleasure, and there will be no undertaking of the long conative train involved in the care and rearing of a family. Thus, while it would appear that a life " devoted to pleasure " is in fact made up of the pursuit of various instinctive ends in easy forms, yet it is easy to see how an agent could come to think of that which unites them all and gives value to the whole as constituted by the element of pleasure.

It has been maintained that it is a case of pleasure being made the end of action when, as sometimes happens, a man takes deliberate steps to create a want or appetite, solely with the end, as supposed, of obtaining the pleasure of satisfying it. A man who has lost his appetite for food takes exercise with the object of recreating it, or an epicure takes drugs or stimulants of various kinds in order to stimulate the taste satisfactions of certain foods and drinks. It is hardly true to say that the object in such cases as these is primarily the pleasure in the acute form obtained at the moment of satisfying the appetite. The primary object is rather to restore that sense of the goodness of life which is found, as we have seen, in the alternation, within due limits, of want and satisfaction. The life passed on one level is experienced as monotonous and depressed, and there is effort to restore the life to a higher level of consciousness.[1] It would be possible to describe this as an impulse towards the fulness of conscious life rather than towards pleasure. But it would seem that in fact, in so far as the present cases are concerned, the amount of pleasure and the degree of intensity or fulness of the conscious life go together. Life is more pleasant, and also more intensely lived, when there is the normal alternation of want and satisfaction. In striving to live more fully there is also striving towards more pleasure. And it is possible that in a mind able to conceive of pleasure separately there may also be some idea that therein lies the value of the whole process. Moreover, inasmuch

[1] Cf. McDougall, *Outline of Psychology*, 271, on this point.

as pleasure is undoubtedly at its highest at the moment when the pre-existent craving is satisfied, it is possible that, in thinking of the pleasantness of the process, the agent will pay regard especially to that moment.

A further complication occurs when we hesitate between alternative ends. Holding the two together in idea, we can compare the amount of the pleasure to be anticipated in each case. We ask ourselves " Which shall I enjoy the most ? " This is the way in which we actually decide many doubtful questions, and it is the easiest way of doing so. It must be plain that even here the anticipated pleasure does not constitute the main part of the driving force. The amount of the pleasure depends on the strength of the respective instinctive impulses which are to be satisfied by the ends. Hence the comparison, though consciously made in terms of pleasure, is really between the strength of the competing impulses, which constitute the driving force in either direction. But though this remains true in the simple cases in which only the intensity of pleasure is the ground of comparison, it must be qualified for those cases into which other considerations enter. We are often motived not by the strongest impulse or intensest pleasure, but by ideas of the duration and number of satisfactory moments of life which will be secured by alternative courses of action. We ask ourselves whether, if we follow a present strong impulse promising intense pleasure, we may not sacrifice other pleasant experiences each individually less intense, but spread over a much longer period. Here it is plain the decision is governed not by the strength of the competing impulses, but by an abstract consideration of the amount of value. This consideration, at a stage of fairly developed intellect, can govern and control the effects of instinctive impulses, even though it does not supply the original driving force.

There is a certain difference between the instincts of bodily maintenance and reproduction and on the other hand the impulse to self-maximation through power, which we may look at in this connection. The former are from

the first directed towards objective ends, and the feeling
going with them is a secondary matter. We have seen
how there emerges from the will to maintenance of the
course of the bodily sensations by insensible gradations
a will towards the intensification of consciousness,
towards a higher level of consciousness. With this process
of development it is the conscious state of the agent,
the feeling of elation, which appears as the valuable
end sought. This state is only attained by means of
objective change, i.e. by bringing about the situation of
dominance of the self over external force. But in bringing
this about it is rather the subjective condition, the feeling,
which comes to be recognized as valuable. The action is
increasingly directed towards bringing about a state of
the self, regarded as valuable. From the first this element
in the motive must be more prominent than with the
other instinctive impulses.

Thus it is no doubt true that there is in the feelings
no original force that leads to action. The source of all
movement and action lies in the driving force of the main
instincts, that is to say in the inherent energy of the
organism striving towards outlet in the forms prescribed
by its inherited structure. The feelings of pleasure and
unpleasure are secondary results dependent on the successful or unsuccessful working of these instincts. Yet,
in the more advanced intellectual stages of which we have
been speaking, it would not be true to say that pleasure
remains a superfluous addition, and that action would
be quite the same whether it was there or not. The action
which consists in the working out of an instinctive impulse
is also in fact that which brings about the greatest
amount of pleasure. In the course of pursuing some
instinctive train of activity, it is possible for those who,
however obscurely, have formed the idea that value and
pleasure coincide to sustain and confirm their action to
some extent by the thought of the pleasantness, and to
look forward to the attainment of some ultimate end as
especially pleasurable. As some writers of the hedonistic

T

school have pointed out, we can alternate between attention to the objective ends which are being pursued and to the " subjective " or feeling side of the experience.[1] At times in the midst of objective pursuit we can turn round on ourselves and reflect on the experience as pleasurable. The feeling becomes temporarily an object in the sense that we give ourselves up to it ; and it is recognized that it is this which gives value to the total activity. Thus the pleasure can become what Aristotle described as " that which completes the activity of life as a supervening end ".[2] This conscious recognition of pleasure as " good " and of unpleasure as " bad " is, we shall be inclined to conclude, based on the fact that it is only in pleasure and unpleasure that the element of value is added to the success or non-success of conations. Thus there is constituted what we might term a " secondary " or psychological acceptance of pleasant experience and rejection of unpleasant experience, based on the fact of felt value, positive or negative as the case may be.

The above account not only gives, it may be hoped, a true picture of what happens in desire, but also enables us to see how easily the theory could arise that pleasure and unpleasure are the sole objects of desire and aversion. It would certainly be strange if a theory so widely held and so often defended as self-evident had not some substantial basis in fact. The first reason to be given for the formation of this theory is found in the fact that craving frequently exists in a subconscious form. In the case of an unexpected sensory pleasure, such as a taste or smell, inasmuch as the subject was not fully conscious beforehand of the craving of the sense organ, it would probably appear to him as though the pleasure came first and the conation to maintain it was its consequence. He will be likely to use such language as " I wanted to retain that sensation because I found it pleasant ".

---

[1] See Bain, *Emotions and the Will*, 437, and Sidgwick, *Methods of Ethics*, 51, who speaks of an " alternating rhythm ".

[2] Aristotle, *Ethics*, X, 4, 8.

When the recurrence of the sensation is suggested, it is likely to seem to him as though it was the idea of the pleasure of the experience which awakened craving and desire *e nihilo*. Similarly unpleasant sensory experience as such will seem to be the cause of aversion. In those cases where the pleasant experience is normally preceded by a conscious craving, e.g. in the satisfaction of hunger, it is not so likely that the impulse will be thought of as desire for pleasure. Ordinary thought and language will be more inclined to recognize that the pleasure is dependent on the pre-existing craving. But still, in order to create an agreement between this and the first-mentioned class of case, it is possible that the impulse towards food may be spoken of as aversion from the unpleasure of hunger and desire for the pleasure of eating. If again we take an instinctive impulse such as that of ambition, we see that it is often the case that in the history of the individual mind the pursuit does not come consciously first. In the development of the child situations of dependence on others occur, and a sense of inferiority accompanied by unpleasure is aroused; and on the other hand the experience of mastery and heightened self-feeling occurs in such situations as relations to other children or its own toys and unexpected praise from elders, and is accompanied by pleasure. The experience may be pleasant or unpleasant, as the case may be, though there has been no conscious striving beforehand towards power and heightened self-feeling. The reason is that the instinct is at first latent and subconscious and only awakens gradually into full consciousness. So too the existence of sexual love may first be betrayed in the consciousness of the agent by feelings of pleasure and unpleasure. The feelings, having occurred first, may appear as the starting point of the process. The second reason for the formation of the hedonist theory lies in the idea of the identity of pleasure and value, an idea which, as we have seen, comes naturally to be held by the mind capable of abstraction and reflection, and has indeed much to be said for it. That which is conceived of as possessing value is also thought of as that which is sought for its own sake, and the possibility is ignored that pleasure is originally and essentially something which comes unsought and superadded to the activity of life.

It is advisable now to give a somewhat fuller account of what happens when through experiences of success and failure it is learnt what actions bring about desired ends. For it has been supposed that it is the feelings of pleasure and unpleasure which confirm or " stamp in " these actions. The question is now of the means to desired ends, not of actions or ends valuable in themselves. We may, it is hoped, find that the views taken herein throw some light on the disputed questions of purpose and adaptation in conduct.

The simplest form of action exists where there is direct impulse to exercise on the part of the organism. The muscles crave exercise, and this leads directly to discharge in movement which satisfies the need. The question of adapted conduct is somewhat more complex. It asks how, given some unfulfilled impulse to activity or other disturbance of equilibrium on the sensory side (proceeding from either internal or external cause), the organism finds the movement adapted to fulfil that tendency and restore equilibrium. It asks, in other words, how some need originating in the sensory neurones passes into the appropriate and successful motor reaction. With animals, even those very low in the scale of intelligence, who can have no explicit memory-ideas, it is found that there is learning as the result of successful action. A crayfish placed in a pen, which has two passages, one a blind alley and the other allowing free exit to water, at first tries both directions impartially ; but after a number of experiences of escape, learns to go almost invariably straight for the open passage.[1] Many similar experiments have

---

[1] Jennings, *Behaviour of Lower Organisms*, 255 and 256, quoting Yerkes and Huggins.

been performed with animals. Cats, for instance, have been placed in cages from which escape to food is possible only by some unusual action, such as pulling a loop or depressing a lever. The first result is random struggle and movements. One of these accidentally opens the cage. Thereafter this successful movement is performed with gradually increasing frequency when the animal is again put in the cage.

Let us in the first place for the sake of simplicity give a sketch in a purely schematic form of what we can believe to be the underlying neural facts in these cases. A certain group of sensory neurones in the organism requires adequate excitation by the appropriate stimulus. In the absence of such stimulation they will be in a state of tension or craving. We will call this group of neurones SC. There is at first no ready-màde associative connection bringing about a movement which leads to the resolution of the tension. The consequence is general restless movement of the whole organism, a series of innervations of motor elements, which we may designate MA, MB, MC. None of these terminate the tension, which thus continues unabated or increases. In the course of the random movements one, which we may call MR, does by accident bring about a satisfaction of the craving of SC, by enabling it to exercise that complete form of activity towards which it was striving. The activity of SC thereupon ceases for the time, and therewith also the tension and restlessness of the organism. On the next occasion when SC is again in a state of craving, and the general cognitive situation is approximately the same, the animal does not repeat the movements of MA, MB, MC exactly as before. It has at least a bias to proceed direct to MR, and this eventually after sufficient repetitions it always does. If we assimilated the process to that of other ordinary association, i.e. the tendency to repeat the same movements in the same order as before on a given cue being provided, a process similar to the formation of a habit, undoubtedly with the repetition there would arise a tendency to repeat MA, MB, MC, etc., more rapidly and efficiently, and perhaps even to some extent to telescope them together ; but it is difficult to see how any tendency could arise to cut them out altogether and proceed direct to MR. The excitation of SC would only act as the cue releasing a series of movements, which would continue as long as the excitation of SC continued ; and when one of the movements happened to terminate that excitation, then automatically of course it would also put an end to the continuance of further movement resulting from SC. The only possible explanation of the facts of shortening seems to me to be based on the fact that the activity of SC is throughout of a nature that needs and strives towards a future end, that it is seeking for something to satisfy its need. That movement therefore which immediately provides the end, which passes directly into the experience of satisfaction, becomes associated with the craving activity of SC as bringing that which is needed and satisfying. We must remember that the movement MR can hardly be cut off as quite separate from the moment of satisfaction. It either is in immediate contact with the moment of satisfaction, passing directly into it, or else it continues during the process of satisfaction, being the means by which the process is sustained and the satiety term reached. In the latter case the craving energy of SC continues, in a diminishing degree, throughout, and is experienced as activating MR, as is obvious from the fact that, if external impediment to the movement MR arises before satiety is reached, craving is again strongly awakened, and passes into a vigorous effort towards the reinstatement of MR. The result is that MR forms an associative connection with SC of a quite special character. It appears as that which satisfies the impulse of SC, and thus as that which is specially adapted to the satisfaction of SC as right and proper. On subsequent occasions when a generally similar situation occurs, if MA, MB, MC occur, they will occur without that special connection, with something that we can only

describe as a sense of " wrongness ", whereas in contrast
MR will occur with a sense of " rightness ". The tendencies to movements MA, etc., will be cut off at the start,
and the tension of SC will discharge into MR with a
sense of satisfaction and a special energy. SC, inasmuch as
it is throughout striving towards the future, is capable of
forming a connection with any movement ensuing from
it ; but it will have formed a connection of a unique
and preferential character with the movement which is
associated with satisfaction. This must be a connection
quite different in character from any formed between
sensations and movements by the mere force of repetition.
In this account there is no need to assume the existence
of explicit ideas of the future, either of the end of
satisfaction, or of MR as the movement required. We
have however every right to assume some consciousness
in all these cases. An impulse or craving which strives
towards the future must of its own intrinsic nature always
yield some awareness of the direction in which satisfaction is to be found. With this there must naturally
go also some awareness of the progress being made at the
moment as either in the direction of the needed end, or
not in the direction, and therewith a slight feeling either
of pleasure or unpleasure. No more than this amount
of consciousness need be assumed by the account given.
Longer trains of association can be formed in the same
way. A movement or a sensation which brings MR
nearer or makes it more possible comes also to share in the
sense of rightness already acquired by MR ; but it is
obvious that mere precedence in time is not enough.
In order to be felt as " right " in direction and to obtain
this preferential selection, the movement or the sensation
must be experienced as that which brings nearer or progressively reinstates MR.

   To apply this simple scheme in a concrete case must
naturally be difficult because there is behind any concrete
case a complex history of racial development, the full
details of which cannot possibly be known to us. We

may however attempt a sketch on the above lines of what happens in the commonest case, that of food seeking. When food is eaten there is a satisfaction given to the craving of various sensory nervous elements towards adequate activity, for the most part those which mediate organic sensations, but also those which mediate taste. These correspond to the " SC " nervous elements, as described above. Simultaneously there are various sensations of other organs, those of contact, sight, and smell, which we may call ST, SV, SO. At the same time there are also occurring the activities of a whole group of motor neurones, as well as of secretory organs, in the main those of lips, tongue, throat, etc., concerned in the ingestion of the food. As we know them, these activities occur as apparently immediate reflexes, brought about by the tension activity of SC, and the sensations ST, SV, SO. But if the general view taken here has any correctness, it is natural to believe that these movements have themselves been learnt as that which satisfies the craving of SC by bringing about a full form of its activity, and that they have thus acquired an immediate connection of " rightness " in connection with the activity of SC. The craving energy of SC tends to discharge immediately into the channels of these movements, as those which procure the needed end, and they continue into the period of satisfaction, sustaining it and making it possible. To use the expression usual in discussions on the subject, they constitute the consummatory response. They correspond to what we previously called MR. ST, SV, and SO have also formed a connection with SC as the accompaniment and sign of satisfaction. Given these connections formed by previous experience of food taking, it may be assumed that SV and SO occur by themselves on another occasion, as distance perceptions of the food object, when SC is already in a state of craving, perhaps slight. The first result will be a discharge of energy into the channels of MR, the group of consummatory responses. But actual satisfaction of the craving will not follow, and tension and restlessness will extend so as to cause movements of the whole organism. Among these movements may be some leading either to or from the object. But those leading away from the object would diminish the intensity of SV and SO, whereas those leading towards it will progressively restore those sensations to an identity with that form in which they are associated with the consummatory response and the full satisfaction of SC. The sensations going with approach to the object will therefore be experienced as increasingly " right ", and the organism will draw towards the object with increasing energy, until the consummatory response is possible. In the same way a chain of actions and sensations leading backwards in an increasing length from the end terms of the consummatory response and the satisfaction can be established, even without the aid of explicit memory-ideas. The series to an increasing extent can share in the qualities originally belonging to the end terms. But of course as explicit ideas are formed, the range of such purposive trains can be greatly increased.

It would seem to me that any theory on this subject which does not recognize a fundamentally purposive character in the governing neural activity cannot give an adequate picture of the facts. In a recent article, " The Neural Basis of Purposive Activity ",[1] G. C. Grindley gives an account which may be summarized as follows. When an animal is hungry there is active a powerful group of neurones (stomachic, etc.) which through the inherited structure bring about certain movements ; walking, scratching, pecking at small objects, by the chick, are the examples given. The active group of neurones, called by him the E neurones, corresponds to what we termed above " SC ". Through the medium of the movements mentioned there is progress towards a consummatory response (swallowing), which brings the behaviour cycle to an end, probably because at this moment the

[1] *British Journal of Psychology*, October 1927, 180–2.

whole energy of the SC (or E) neurones is discharged into this response, and so they remain quiescent for a time afterwards. Suppose that a chick has several times been placed in a position where it gets food by turning to the right, and not by turning to the left, it learns to go more often to the right and so get the food. The supposition made to account for this is that, when the discharge of energy takes place from SC to the consummatory response, SC is also able at the same moment to form an associative connection with the movement (turning to the right) which has immediately preceded the discharge, and that this connection can become so strong and intimate that in future the excitation of SC will directly activate the neurones concerned in turning to the right (which we call for shortness B neurones). But admittedly this supposition needs justification. If the discharge of SC into the consummatory response has only taken place after the activity of B, what would normally happen is that in future B would tend to activate the discharge of SC and not vice versa ; and the supposition that a reverse connection is somehow formed appears somewhat arbitrary. As the result of the experiments of Wohlgemuth, there is at least strong reason for the belief that associations between movements, formed ordinarily through contiguity and repetition, only operate in the one direction and cannot be reversed.[1] If ABC movements have occurred in that order before, A will suggest B in future but not vice versa. In the cases now under consideration however it is plain that connections *are* formed in the reverse direction. A movement which has led to the consummatory response does actually acquire a meaning and value from that fact ; and this influence can be extended backwards for some distance over a series of movements. The only possible explanation seems to be that there is something itself purposive in the neural basis of conscious purposive activity. Only that which is, in its degree,

[1] See *British Journal of Psychology* (1912–13), Vol. 5, p. 465.

purposive could be capable of the preferential selection
of that movement which has preceded and led up to the
fulfilment of the purpose. This would be only in accordance with the view, expressed by many philosophers,
that to purpose conceived as a reference to the future
there can be no purely material correlate, possessing
only movement of a mechanical order.

Negative learning, i.e. the acquisition of movements
adapted to avoid the harmful and unpleasant, is often
regarded as requiring a further explanation, different from
that of positive learning, i.e. the acquisition of movements
to obtain the beneficial and pleasant.[1] The example
usually quoted is that of the burnt child who dreads the
fire. A young child who has, following its instinctive
impulse to grasp at a bright object, put its hand into a
flame, and then withdrawn it hastily when burnt, learns
in future to inhibit the grasping reaction in face of a
flame. The simple explanation given of this is often as
follows : After the child has been burnt, on the next
occasion the sight of the flame reinstates incipiently the
tendency, not only to the grasping reaction, but also to
the avoiding reaction, and as they cannot take place
simultaneously, there is a tendency for the stronger, the
avoiding reaction, to prevail. This complication of response goes parallel with a complication in respect of
cognition. The object is perceived simultaneously as
visually bright and with the suggestion also of " pain
producing ", just as, when we have touched an object,
it gives us in future simultaneously the sensation of
colour (e.g. redness) and an impression of hardness.
To the unitary object there corresponds a unitary reaction. This is practically in accordance with the account
on physiological lines given by James.[2] Whether it
can be accepted depends, I think, on much the same
considerations as those applicable to " positive " learning.
The two sets of facts are not really distinct. It may sound

[1] E.g. by Grindley, in the article quoted above.
[2] *Principles of Psychology*, II, 590–1.

plausible at first sight to say that, two incompatible reactions being impossible towards a single object, that only is carried out which is the strongest, and that the conflict and suppression can take place intra-cerebrally, so that no trace of the inhibited reaction would appear in outward movement. But even if we confine ourselves to the simple sort of case mentioned, it can be seen that this is very improbable. There is no necessary competition and incompatibility between the two reactions, grasping and withdrawing, provided, as on the first occasion, they again take place successively. The pain experience on the first occasion only occurred via the grasping movement, and if the grasping movement brought about a sensation, either indifferent or satisfying some other instinctive need, of which the further action of withdrawal were the indifferent or pleasant expression, then the more often the series were repeated, the stronger would be the tendency always to repeat it in the same order. The most we should expect in that case would be an increase in the rapidity with which the reactions followed, which might lead to a sort of merging or telescoping. We should *not* expect that after one or very few repetitions, as actually often happens, there should be a total suppression of the one response and a complete victory of the other.[1] Hobhouse recognizes that, in order to account for this immediate confirmation or inhibition of responses, recourse must be had to the effects of feeling (pleasure

---

[1] J. B. Watson has had the courage to experiment with a child and a flame. He states that 150 trials were necessary in order to perfect the tendency to withdrawal (*Psychology from the Standpoint of a Behaviourist*, 300). But such an experiment can hardly be accepted as a fair test, because in no single instance could the child be allowed to burn itself seriously; and measures were taken to avoid this. Probably, too, at the age of the child (150 to 220 days) any sort of learning was slow and difficult. According to Lloyd Morgan, a chick sometimes learns to avoid pecking at the cinnabar caterpillar after one attempt (*Habit and Instinct*, 41). As another instance of an animal low in the scale of adaptability, Dahl found that, when a spider was given a fly dipped in turpentine, it avoided attacking the fly after three attempts (quoted by Hobhouse, *Mind in Evolution*, 117). A number of similar facts can be found given by Piéron, *Evolution de la Mémoire*, 125–9.

or unpleasure), or at least to the psycho-physical process in which feeling is involved.[1] But this in itself does not carry us very far, unless we are prepared to assume the causal efficacy of feeling at very low stages of mental development; and this it seems very difficult to do. A more explicit meaning is however given to these supposed effects of feeling in the recognition of the fact that a conational process, such as that of grasping at a bright object, is essentially a unitary whole directed towards an end. It is aimed at the obtaining of a tactual sensation. That which contradicts or disappoints this end by the fact of yielding a pain sensation accompanied by an avoiding reaction, must thereby establish a relation with the conation as a whole and so in future tend to inhibit it. There is, as it might be expressed, an anticipatory sensation in the grasping effort; and thus the visual sensation which suggests a contradiction or disappointment of the prospective tactual sensation cuts off the total conative effort at the start.[2] The account thus given is certainly true as far as it goes. But it cannot be accepted as giving a complete account of all the facts. It does give a complete account of those cases where the agent learns to modify or suppress an originally instinctive reaction because of experiences of non-success; for example, where the agent after repeated attempts to grasp at a certain sort of object, say a shadow, learns to desist because of non-attainment of a tactual sensation. But in the case before us it is obvious that the pain experience is something more than a disappointment of the grasping impulse. It is something in regard to which there is aversion and avoidance apart from any preceding impulse to grasp. It appears as " bad " or " to be avoided " in itself, and this fact certainly plays an important part in the learning. Thus, if we consider the matter further, it will, I think, be obvious that we have to account, not

---

[1] Hobhouse, *Mind in Evolution*, 118, and *Development and Purpose*, 64.

[2] See Hobhouse, *Mind in Evolution*, 122. Stout, *Manual of Psychology*, 187–90. Perry, *General Theory of Value*, 188–9.

only for the case mentioned above, in which a grasping impulse towards the bright object is suppressed owing to the pain experience, but also for that case in which a flame (or other harmful object) is by some external agency or by accident brought in contact with the body of the living being, and the living being thereupon learns to avoid it in future. In such cases the visual (or other distance) effects of the object come to be treated as a warning of danger. It seems to be the case that living beings learn to avoid harmful and disagreeable objects more readily when there is in the first place, as the result of an instinctive impulse, some tendency to approach and seize them.[1] Nevertheless animals also learn to avoid, through distance effects, harmful objects with which they have come in contact accidentally or through external agency. The dog quickly learns to shrink at the sight of the whip. We can then hardly answer the question before us without asking what is the inner nature of the conative impulse to withdrawal, which is thus reinstated by the distance effects of the object. According to the account already given by us,[2] this avoidance is the result of an automatic reaction by the nervous elements primarily affected, which becomes for the whole organism an effort to restore the normal course of the vital processes as against incipient depression or disturbance. There is a constant underlying will of the self directed towards the maintenance of the vital activity, a fact shown in the conscious aversion and unpleasure which immediately arise from disturbance or depression, and the fear which goes with the onset and increase of depression. While there is always a possibility that, when one experience follows another closely, an associative connection may be formed such that the first may be treated as a sign of the second, a specially close connection is likely to be formed where the second experience is of a harmful character. In striving towards future

---

[1] This seems to follow from the experiments of Yerkes and Schaeffer, quoted by Hobhouse, *Mind in Evolution*, 123.

[2] See pp. 50 and 51.

self-maintenance, in its latent semi-defensive and watchful attitude which is constantly present, the mind is
prepared at all times to treat individual sensations as
signs either of future success or of future failure. That
which has once, or oftener, passed immediately into the
experience of obstructed vital activity can quickly become
a warning sign of it and provoke by anticipation the
avoiding effort accompanied by aversion. The mind
will of itself on the appearance of the sign leap forward at
once to the attitude of avoidance and aversion. By itself
however, at anything except a somewhat highly developed
stage of intellect, this fact could only cause the immediate antecedent of the unpleasant experience, that
which has passed directly into it, to become the sign of it
in future. For instance, in the case of a flame being
brought close to the hand, or indeed any other part of the
child's body, the warmth sensation could thus become a
sign of burning pain to come and give the cue for avoidance. It is here we reach the further part played in the
matter by the pre-existing impulse to grasp at the bright
object. It helps to bind the total experience into a unitary
whole for the subject. The impulse to grasp at the bright
object is directed towards an end, that of obtaining
tactual sensations in the hand, for which there is a craving.
The end which normally closes this train of action, i.e.
the tactual sensation, becomes linked to it with a more
or less definite expectation. If another sort of sensation,
itself of a vivid and interesting character, that of burning,
results from the movement, it will become the expected
end of the grasping impulse when directed towards a
particular sort of bright visual object. Thus the fact
that the bright object is already a cause of attention and
interest to the child will have the result of making it
possible for the warning to operate from further off.
The bright visual object becomes an easily recognized
signal of harm, and the agent is likely to become aware
of the danger at an earlier point of action than if the
object did not from the first arouse attention and interest.

We have taken as our example in the foregoing a very simple case of learning a single successful reaction. The conclusions drawn are even more plainly confirmed by those cases in which the living being in a harmful situation tries several methods of escape until it finds a successful one, and acquires the capacity, when the same situation recurs later, to suppress the unsuccessful methods and proceed direct to the successful reaction. This fact is found to exist almost throughout the animal world.[1] It is obvious that here no theory of the effect of mere repetition is sufficient to account for the facts. It must be believed that there is a governing factor, the effort of the living being towards the re-establishment of its normal life, which brings about the suppression of the unsuccessful reactions. This governing factor corresponds to the craving impulse of what in the case of " positive " learning we called the " SC " neurones. The random struggles to obtain food correspond precisely to those directed towards escape from a present harmful situation and restoration of normal bodily conditions. The principles governing " negative " and " positive " learning are in fact the same.

It is natural to ask here what is the part played in conduct by ideas, and particularly ideas of movement. The view of James was that primarily all movements are reflex, instinctive or emotional, and must be performed without prevision, and that in order to perform a voluntary movement, which is a secondary and derived phenomenon, memory-images of previous involuntary movements are requisite. " Whether or no there be anything else in the mind at the moment when we consciously will a certain act, a mental conception made up of memory-images of these sensations (i.e. of movement), defining which special act it is, must be there."[2] We can agree

[1] Vide the well-known experiment of Jennings with Stentor, a unicellular organism (*Behaviour of the Lower Organisms*, 174–7). The same has been found with other lowly organisms.
[2] James, *Principles of Psychology*, II, 492.

that this question is one affecting in the first place what is a matter of means not of ends. The prime mover, we would say, is the will of the organism to act out its impulse to life. This is expressed immediately in some movements to which there is a direct tendency. When an impediment to the exercise of any form of vital activity is met with, it is expressed by tension, random movement, and trial and error, until a successful movement is hit on. The only question that would seem to arise is whether, when a movement has thus been found, it is necessary, in order that it may be voluntarily carried out again, that there should precede it ideas of the movement in the form of kinæsthetic and visual sensations. But observation has tended to show that ideas of the movement to be voluntarily performed are sometimes, but by no means always, present beforehand. When a more or less definite idea is present before a movement, it is rather the idea of the effect to be produced. Given that a desired result has been obtained by a certain movement before, it would seem that the movement can be reproduced by the idea of the result, and by a general idea of the nature of the movement required, the sensations of the actual detailed movement, as it proceeds, appearing with a certain sense of " rightness ".[1] More definite ideas of the movement, in the form both of kinæsthetic and visual images, are likely to appear if there is some external impediment which prevents the movement being carried out at once. It must however be admitted that introspection on the point in question is a matter of some difficulty and doubt.

The question of " ideo-motor " action as ordinarily conceived is somewhat different from that discussed above. It is the question how far ideas, whether of movements to be performed or of results to be brought about, ever actually constitute the motive force for conduct, apart from any other impulse or desire. It is of course

[1] Cf. Woodworth, *Psychology ; a Study of Mental Life*, 524-8, on this point.

U

obvious that the mere will to act out an idea, to translate
it into reality, is not the ultimate principle of action.
That is found in the self-maintaining effort of the living
being, as expressed in the various instincts. But sometimes undoubtedly the mere suggestion of a movement
does result in its performance. As we saw in discussing
altruistic sympathy and æsthetic sympathy (see pp. 188
and 226–7) the idea of a movement carries with it, perhaps
always, some incipient innervation of the muscles concerned in the movement. This may pass into the actual
performances of the movement, provided there is at the
moment no other impulse to action derived from an instinctive need of the agent's own. The simplest and commonest form of this sort of action is that which appears
as automatic and semi-mechanical imitation of others.
Some persons are no doubt more open to such suggestions
than others, having less force of individual impulse ;
and all are no doubt more suggestible at some times than
at others.

With this simplest form of the ideo-motor impulse
we may contrast another which is more complex and can
only appear in highly developed minds. Its condition
again is that there is present in the agent no strong
instinctive need, either because his needs are easily
satisfied for him without active effort of his own, or
because there is no material on which he can exercise
himself in any form of play. In this state the active
mind must feel the need for some change of content.
This need can sometimes be satisfied for a time by the
play of images ; but such satisfaction does not as a rule
last long. The conscious life of mind is only fully maintained over against objects possessing the vividness
and force of sensory presentation. Images fail to satisfy
by reason of their lack of vividness and impressional
force. Hence the conscious life loses in intensity and
seems to descend to a lower level when there is no change
of external objective content. It is in these circumstances that there arises a desire for mere change for its

own sake. If the idea of some movement or action is suggested somehow to such a vacant and dissatisfied mind, it may carry it out as the first and most obvious means of effecting a change of content. This may not occur very often. But we can see that, when it does, it exemplifies the most fundamental need of mind, that to maintain the level of its conscious existence. We can hardly describe it as due to the impulsive force of ideas as such. It is probable that sometimes this motive and the impulse to mechanical imitation may coincide and reinforce each other.

We can from the point of view now reached deal with a subsidiary question, which has often been discussed in regard to pleasures and unpleasures, particularly those of sensory origin. This is the so-called relativity of feelings. We all know that, if we have been suffering from a severe toothache, and it decreases notably, though still persisting in the lessened form, the resulting state will probably be for a time experienced as pleasant, though if it had occurred after an indifferent or pleasant state it would have been unpleasant. Again, a sweet taste, which would be pleasant if it occurred after a state of indifference, may be slightly unpleasant after a much stronger sensation of sweetness. It is obvious that to appeal to a so-called general law of contrast is meaningless. To take the case of unpleasure first, we find that Lehmann, in discussing the question, gives an explanation on physiological lines.[1] According to him the assimilation tendencies, set up by the reaction to the original stimulus causing the intense unpleasure, still continue when the stimulus decreases, and so are able to make good the dissimilation due to the lessened stimulation. It is possible that there may be some truth in this, i.e. that protective mechanisms set in action by an intense stimulus still continue for a time when the stimulus decreases. But this

---

[1] Lehmann, *Die Hauptgesetze des menschlichen Gefühlslebens*, 255–7.

involves a number of hypothetical factors. It seems to me we are on surer ground if we look for an explanation rather in conscious factors. During the period of intense unpleasure, the mind was striving to terminate the existing state of bodily sensation with its accompanying feeling. A diminution of the unpleasant sensations appears as a partial satisfaction of this striving. Inasmuch as it is a partial fulfilment of a conation, a move at least in the required direction, it must appear as pleasant. Moreover this relief and satisfaction of the mental impulse seem to point the way to a complete cessation of the unpleasant conditions, and this opens the door to hope. If however the unpleasant sensation persists for some time in its diminished degree, the effect of the initial sense of relief soon dies away and the sensation becomes unpleasant again. This seems in accordance with our ordinary experience. If we turn to the parallel cases of pleasure, it is obvious that a stimulus on repetition may cease to cause pleasure ; and this must be due to some fatigue condition of the sense organ concerned. There are however cases in which this explanation cannot suffice. Lehmann gives the following as an instance.[1] We eat the first strawberries of the season with great pleasure, even if not quite ripe. The pleasure may increase for a time as the strawberries get riper. But after a little time it gets less, and towards the end of the season we may be comparatively indifferent in the matter. This cannot be due to any fatigue or adaptation of the taste organs ; for such a condition would not last over from one day to another. In this sort of case again we must, as Lehmann indeed says, appeal to central factors, those involving in some degree the conscious self. The pleasure of eating the first strawberries is a complex one, depending partly on the sensory craving for a certain combination of taste and odour sensations, partly on the fact that this combination not having been experienced for some time the memory-images of it are

---

[1] Lehmann, op. cit., 258–60.

relatively faint, and so, when it occurs, it carries with it something of the interest and excitement of novelty.[1] It is this second factor which diminishes with repetition of the experience. The taste and flavour combination becomes more familiar, and whenever the fruit is seen or suggested, it is called up more readily in the form of images. With this clear anticipation the interest of the actual eating experience grows less, in so far as it depended on the attraction of novelty ; and so too the keenness of desire for the experience will diminish. In this we find again an example in which the more or less conscious memory of the value of an experience has an effect on desire. It seems clear that the facts in a case like this must be dependent on some central factors such as those mentioned. Mere repetition of a stimulus would appear to have different effects in different cases, so far as the purely physiological side is concerned. Sometimes through repetition the need of the sense organ for the stimulus is increased ; and craving can thus be induced and become stronger. This happens in many cases of what we called acquired tastes. Sometimes the constant repetition of the stimulus causes satiety and disgust. I do not think we know what are the total physiological facts which cause the difference in these two classes of case.

[1] We shall deal later with the nature of the value of novelty.

PART VI

OTHER KINDS OF FEELING. THE PSYCHOLOGY OF VALUES

WE have defined pleasure and unpleasure as mental elements accompanying certain forms of the mental process, pleasure being that which goes with success, effectiveness, and smooth working, unpleasure that which goes with failure and obstructed working. It seems antecedently improbable that there should be no other forms taken by the mental functioning, with which there are connected separate elements as feelings. We shall see, I think, that we can classify the forms of the mental processes in other ways than under the heading of " success " or " non-success ". While viewed from outside these can be termed forms of the mental functioning, from inside they must be designated as states or affections of the self, in some case an " attitude " of the self, in others a passive condition of the self. There does not seem to be a suitable term in English to describe these " self-states ". In German the term *Bewusstseinslage* seems to denote what is here intended, i.e. a state or condition of consciousness.[1] The question which we shall have to discuss is whether to all or any of these mental attitudes or states there is added the element of feeling, i.e. that element of warmth and intimacy in respect of which there is a movement between degrees of value and non-value, as we have found with pleasure and unpleasure. It seems not impossible that a mental attitude or *Bewusstseinslage*

---

[1] This term is used by Orth, *Gefühl und Bewusstseinslage*, 69–75. But his definition is not very clear.

should exist without necessarily carrying with it any sort of feeling.

There is in the first place a group of mental attitudes, in which we have the forms taken by the purely cognitive response to objects. We have assumed in this work that all conscious experience takes place in the form of " subject-perceiving object ". There is thus a fundamental form of the affection of the subject, which always exists in mental life, that in respect of which objects appear as other than, and given to or imposed upon, the subject. Lipps describes this as the " immediate symptom of consciousness for the fact that something foreign to the unity of my mental life, not born of it, comes against this unity and breaks into it ".[1] This most fundamental form of subjective attitude exists not only in relation to external objects, but also in relation to images, inasmuch as these must always be given to the subject through some process either of association or perseveration, not wholly under the control of the subject. It must always be present, but is subject to differences of degree, being less intense, for example, in the state of æsthetic absorption in an object, than it is when an external object appears as something to be adapted or manipulated for our own purposes. Beyond this we find states of the cognitive subject depending on the relation of the present perception to memory traces left by past impressions. The present object may affect the subject either as different from what has just preceded, or as the same after an interval of difference. In the latter case there is the subjective condition of recognition or familiarity.[2] When mental life is sufficiently advanced for definite memories to exist, expectation of the future is possible, and a given object may appear either as the same or as different to the expected. In the former case the

---

[1] Lipps, *Leitfaden des Psychologie* (1903), 253. The whole of the section on feeling, 249–91, is an attempt to base feeling on the varying forms of subjective attitude.

[2] See pp. 90–1 on recognition as a self-state.

subject is affected by the sense of fulfilment, in the latter by the shock of surprise. Then there are the more complex cognitive attitudes expressed in the various forms of the judgment—affirmation, negation, doubt, supposal, belief, etc. No attempt is made here to give an exhaustive list, but only to give some of the typical forms. If we now ask what is the relation of these attitudes to feeling, we shall see that there are in the first place a number of intellectual attitudes, principally among those last mentioned, such as affirmation and negation, which are never adopted or avoided for their own sake, but always appear as subsidiary means in a conative train directed towards some other end. There can be no element of goodness or badness necessarily attached to any of these attitudes. We find however that there are also forms of intellectual attitude which do seem in themselves to be accompanied by some feeling of value. These are in fact the attitudes involved in the attainment of those ends of the theoretical impulse, the pure impulse to knowledge, which we have already described. Thus the fulfilment of expectation is, apart from other factors, accompanied by a slight tinge of pleasure, because in it the general course of the mental life, with its prospective outlook into the future, runs more smoothly and easily. Orth, taking " doubt " as an example of a *Bewusstseinslage*, examined its connection with feeling under experimental conditions, and came to the conclusion that as a mental state it is not to be classed as itself a feeling, but that feeling may be joined to it as an additional element.[1] He does not give any conclusion as to the nature of the feeling that is joined to the state of doubt. *Primâ facie* it would seem that doubt can never arise unless for some reason the mind has previously been striving towards a decision, aiming at certainty in some form or other, and that therefore it must always yield some awareness of impotence or ineffectiveness, which would mean at least some shade of

[1] Orth, *Gefühl und Bewusstseinslage*, 119–27.

unpleasure. This seems to be confirmed as a rule by the pronouncements of Orth's observers, and ordinary opinion would probably agree as to it. In a few cases it is true Orth's observers do not report unpleasure with the hesitation between alternatives. This no doubt is explicable as follows. In itself the cognitive attitude of hesitation between two alternatives does not include feeling. If we can abstract from any consciousness of the further end, i.e. from our wish to arrive at a decision, and concentrate for the time being on a mere cognitive discussion as to which of two given alternatives may be right, the feeling of unpleasure may temporarily disappear. This presumably happened with Orth's observers. In so far as there is any consciousness that a decision is required or desired, it would seem that unpleasure must accompany the state of doubt. We shall then hold that cognitive attitudes are to be distinguished from the feelings; and that they are only accompanied by feelings of pleasure and unpleasure in so far as they are themselves conative in character, that is to say striving towards that state of mental certainty, ease or power, which is the end of the purely theoretical impulse of curiosity. Such feeling depends on the success or non-success of the conation and is one of pleasure or unpleasure accordingly. It is connected with the conative element and not with the cognitive element as such. It is only a special case of a form taken by the conative response of an instinctive character.

We shall then now ask what are the forms which may be taken by the conative life of the self, as shown in its instinctive impulses, and how feeling is connected with them. It is not intended to refer to the emotions. That which we usually call an emotion, for example fear, anger, or love, is the affective accompaniment going with an instinctive activity, and its character is determined by the character of the instinct, or at least by the particular sort of response which the self is making to the situation of the moment. What we are here asking is whether there are other forms taken by the mental life which yield values parallel to pleasure and unpleasure, and which are capable of applying to different instincts and different sorts of conative response. There are, I would suggest, three forms which the mental life can take, carrying with them feelings which move in degrees of value and non-value, or goodness and badness, as they may be termed. Each of these makes up a " dimension " in which a large number of degrees can exist between the two opposites. These are as follows :

1. The dimension moving between success and failure, effectiveness and non-effectiveness, the smooth and the obstructed working out of the instinctive conations.

2. That moving within degrees of activity and passivity, in respect of which we feel ourselves more or less self-directed.

3. That of the differing depth or intensity with which the conscious self is engaged in the reaction, the result being that the total experience appears on the one hand as in varying degrees, vivid, important, exciting, on the other as deadened, trivial, dull.

1. This has been the subject of the preceding treatment and the endeavour has been to show that on it depends a feeling element which moves between pleasure and unpleasure. No more need be said on this subject here.

2. By degrees of activity and passivity we mean the differences in the extent to which any change in the field of consciousness is felt to be produced by the self. The differences of degree in this respect run through the whole of mental life. In the sphere of external action, with which we will deal first, the minimum of the sense of agency or self-production occurs when the action takes place as the result of automatic association in some form, i.e. when it is induced by mere habit, or by imitation of others or suggestion on the part of others. There is effective in such cases the tendency of a detached system in the mind, working apart from the main stream of the self-maintaining effort of conscious life. The agent either

feels himself passive or, if there is any other conflicting tendency working in him at the moment, feels himself more or less constrained.

In contrast with such actions as these, those actions which spring directly from the will to maintenance of the bodily life, i.e. under the impulsion of a bodily need such as hunger or sex, appear as imposed or compulsory to a lesser degree. It is true that they are performed as a rule as the result of an urge of which the agent himself can give no account, and there is no mental act of consent or fiat. But as expressions of the fundamental will to live and function, they differ, and must be felt to differ, from actions which are the result of some acquired association or of a perseveration. This difference comes out in the case of opposition. An instinctive impulse, when prevented from full exercise, increases in strength and is willed with the full energy of the self. A tendency to action due to mere habit is likely to die out, if prevented from realization. If it recurs and persists, the reason is as a rule some sort of dissociation ; and it is felt as something imposed on the self. It is not sought with persistence and varied effort by the conscious self.

A further form of the same difference may be seen if we compare the impulses of bodily maintenance with that leading to self-maximation. As we have already stated[1] the bodily needs and desires, for a highly conscious being, may appear as something imposed by the necessary physical substratum of life. By contrast, for those capable of making the distinction, the impulse to self-maximation through power means an impulse towards raising the level of the conscious life, and while it appears as springing from the fundamental nature of the self, it also appears as something voluntary and freely adopted, an extra beyond the bare necessity of maintaining what exists. It is perhaps in this point especially that there is a tendency to ascribe a value to the will to power or self-maximation which does not belong to the bodily desires

[1] See pp. 205-6.

and needs. This value of course must pertain to the will to power throughout its course. In so far as it is successful, there is added to it the value of the pleasure going with success.

There is a contrast, arising from similar grounds, to be noted between the activities of play and the serious and whole-hearted pursuit of instinctive ends. This distinction can only be felt by the grown living being, which is capable of serious pursuits. It can hardly exist for the young, who seem to play because they must. For the adult person, who has experience of the serious maintenance of life, there is a consciousness of freedom in any sort of play. It appears as something adopted by him without the drive of any necessity, which can be dropped if desired, and in which he engages with the sense of keeping something in reserve, of sparing to exert his full powers.[1] It is in this point that we are inclined to find a certain value in play as compared with the serious business of life, though as we shall see later there are other considerations which balance this point of superior value.

A consciousness of self-origination appears especially in that more developed form of conduct where there is a choice between alternatives, and the decision is made by any sort of rule, principle or governing end, which the self has adopted and feels as peculiarly its own. In the several experimental studies which have been made of the act of will or choice there is on the whole an agreement that in the moment of decision there is to be detected an awareness of self-activity, which is of quite a special character and to be distinguished from any complex of kinæsthetic and organic sensations.[2] At the same time the investi-

[1] See Groos, *Spiele der Tiere*, 298–9, on this point. As he well points out, there must be some awareness of this sort in the grown dog, which having had experience of serious fighting, sometimes fights playfully.

[2] See Ach, *Ueber den Willensakt und das Temperament*, 239–49. Michotte and Prum, *Le Choix Volontaire*, 193–204. H. M. Wells, *The Phenomenology of Acts of Choice*, 135–45. An opposite view is however maintained by R. H. Wheeler; see his articles quoted by Miss Wells.

gators referred to seem to show a certain vagueness in assigning any antecedent to this " self-activity ", and in analysing it further. It is described in such terms as " designating ", a " mental movement ", or " turning towards ", one of the alternatives ; but a further defini-tion of the content of the mental act seems to be lacking. An activity described as " of the self ", but of which the further antecedents and content cannot be given, would not be a very satisfying conception. Although the general support of the authors mentioned cannot be claimed on this point, it is difficult not to believe that motives are to be found as giving the content of the self-activity which is observed in introspection ; and that it is the motivation which gives the clue to the description of the self-activity. There is some difference between experi-mental studies of this kind and most of our ordinary experiences. The experiments of Michotte and Prum and those of Wells give cases of choice in which sometimes no doubt there might be a sufficient reason for action in the alternatives themselves, but more often the agent would have no sufficient reason for choosing either of the alternatives, apart from the previous instruction given him by the experimenter. These are similar to those cases in ordinary life in which we are presented with two alternatives, one of which has to be taken, but neither of which would urge us to action in itself apart from the given antecedent necessity. The driving force in making the act of choice must therefore be the ante-cedent fact, the decision or the compulsion to take one of the two alternatives instead of doing nothing, which can still influence action though not in the focus of conscious-ness. What yields the consciousness of self-activity in these cases must be the fact that the present act of choice is governed by the previous decision adopted by the self to choose one alternative or the other, instead of taking neither.[1] The results of these experimental obser-

---

[1] I am not sure whether Michotte and Prum would have been in agreement with this. See, however, p. 317, in which they say : " This

vations are noteworthy to us, because they show some consciousness of self-origination even in cases of action where it might have seemed less likely that it would be found. In any case of a decision, where the alternatives are clearly held together in the mind and compared, there must be some motive for preferring the one rather than the other, and the ground of this preference must be capable of being stated as a governing principle, which the self has adopted and by which it governs its actions, though of course there is no need for it to be explicitly formulated in general terms. The clearer however is the consciousness that action in a choice between alternatives is being governed by a reference to the settled principles and character of the self, the stronger will be the sense of self-direction. The agent feels that he is governing his actions by principles adopted into and made part of his settled character ; and in this consciousness there is in general a feeling of a certain value yielded for him. The typical instance of this is the rejection of some bodily gratification or of some sudden impulse of anger because adjudged inconsistent with a man's idea of his social self, i.e. of himself as a member of a community of selves all approximately equal, whose lives he has to respect as they respect his. In this instance an intrinsic value is ascribed to the principle itself. But apart from this there is no doubt that we do find a satisfaction in the mere fact of being ourselves. A value is found in the maintenance of the individual character and personality, and in the sense of independence and self-consistency going therewith, as against other varying impulses or claims which appear to possess some temporary insistent force. The beginnings of this sort of motive seem to appear somewhat early in life. For Stern relates instances in which

act only takes its character of choice by reason of the psychical milieu in which it appears, and notably because it has been preceded by a univocal act deciding the eventual realization of one of the two possibilities before which the subject found himself.'' The nature of the self-activity seems clearer in the acts of will examined by Ach, for they consisted in carrying out a previously adopted decision in opposition to a tendency due to habit.

children, aged about four, have practised what looks like asceticism or voluntary self-control for its own sake, e.g. by deliberately reserving some titbit for a later meal.[1] Undoubtedly asceticism in its later development is largely motived in this way. No doubt it is often the case that the rules of society are obeyed merely out of fear and in a slavish spirit, i.e. as alien and imposed. In such a case the agent will not feel himself as self-determined, and his action will not have for him the value belonging to that consciousness. A form of the same consciousness of agency exists when any purpose is consistently maintained before the mind, and carried out by a prolonged train of action. Some agency is involved in the mere fact of persistently keeping the purpose before one and in resisting distractions. Here too a man feels himself as self-determined.

We can also speak of origination by the self with another meaning. We can mean not so much direction by the self, as creativeness, the production by the self of something new, which is not the mere resultant of past conditions. Every act we perform must have a certain quality of newness. However habitual it may be, it must be an adaptation of what we have learnt to a set of circumstances which is not quite the same as what has preceded. All our acts might therefore be called creative in some degree. But some have more of the quality of newness than others. For example, when we learn any new sort of exercise (skating, dancing, rowing, etc.) we are bringing about something new in respect of ourselves, different from our past actions. And moreover, though we learn by following the pattern set by others, the resultant is an adaptation of the pattern to our own individual body and mind, and must therefore possess some element of actual novelty. In that which we call " invention " it is the same form of novelty or creativeness which is present, but in a much higher degree. That which is " original " must always be based on preceding experience. Origina-

---

[1] Stern, *Psychology of Early Childhood*, 453.

tion without some sort of antecedent pattern does not exist. The originality of an invention consists in the fact that a relation existing in one set of circumstances is, by reason of a point of identity, taken and used in another set. When, for example, the expansive force of steam has been observed, it can be used to pump water or drive vehicles, work previously done by animal power. The originality lies not in the observation of the new fact by itself, which may force itself on the notice ; but firstly in the mere idea of applying it as an intermediary link in a chain of events in place of animal power, the idea that it will fulfil the same function as animal power ; secondly in the analogical adaptation of the existing material (pumps or vehicles) to suit the newly observed force. In order to see that steam can do work, it has to be grasped that a point of identity exists between it and animal power, an idea which seems to come to the mind with something of the nature of a momentary flash of insight. This seen, a new term can be arrived at, i.e. " the expansive force of steam working pumps, or driving vehicles ". The creativeness consists in the " eduction of a correlate " or an " analogical extension ", to use the expressions already quoted from Spearman and Hobhouse.[1] The process has in fact something of the nature of a rule of three sum, in which, however, as the items are something more than mathematical terms, the point of identity which enables the observed relation to be extended to another set of circumstances is not immediately obvious, and is something which the mind seems to grasp in a moment of insight. In a case such as that mentioned the whole process is of course motived by the wish to obtain some result desirable for reasons outside the process itself, some " practical " end, as it would usually be called. But in the mere fact of creativeness, in the sense of having produced something new, it would seem that there does exist a feeling of value for the agent.

[1] See p. 110 above.

x

The example of an invention which we have given above is in fact drawn rather from the sphere of ideas than that of action. Looking further at the sphere of pure ideas, we see that cognitive contents appear as imposed on, or given to, the mind, when they are the result of sense perception or any form of automatically working association. By contrast the general concept appears as something which the mind has sought of its own will. In the sphere of general laws and concepts the mind has raised itself beyond the limits in which it is bound down by the particularity of separate objects, and moves among objects which, though based on particular experiences, are yet in part the result of the mind's own activity. It has freed itself from subservience to the sense particulars and, in order to fulfil its own needs, has mastered and ordered them under general laws. The feeling that goes with this is something more than a pleasure of success. It is a feeling of the superiority in value of the total experience as compared with one limited to individual sense impressions. This element of value seems to be due to the consciousness of self-direction and self-origination.

There may also be new discovery or creation in regard to ideas. But this has in effect been already dealt with in our example of a " practical " invention given above. The only difference is that in speaking of a practical invention we mean one which has as its object the satisfaction of some extraneous need of man ; while in the theoretical sphere the endeavour to discover new laws is made in order to satisfy a purely cognitive need, i.e. the mind's will to find some order in the confusing mass of sense impressions. The method of discovery or invention is the same in both cases, i.e. that of analogical extension.

It might be thought that the value of which we have been speaking here is identical with that yielded by the consciousness of success in attaining power, and is only a sort of pleasure. I think however we are bound to feel that what we have been endeavouring to describe is a feeling not adequately denoted by the word " pleasure ". With successful agency or origination by the self there does no doubt go an element of pleasure. At the same time there is also an element which consists rather in the deepening of the self-consciousness by the sense of self-direction and self-independence. It is the value yielded by my consciousness of being more myself. The opposite to this is rather something privative, a lessened selfhood which exists in the sense of passivity, not the positive non-value of " badness " which is felt when there is unsuccessful effort towards self-assertion. The two elements of value can co-exist, and to some extent fuse, but it is possible to see their difference.

3. It has been our assertion that pleasure, in acute form, occurs when energy which has been striving for discharge obtains free outlet, and that it is greater according as there has been some previous impediment to the discharge. When unused powers are exercised, especially after some repression or impediment, pleasure is high. In these cases the whole level of the conscious life is raised at the same time. The conscious activity seems greater. Pleasure and intensity of conscious life vary together. But even in quite simple experiences we can soon discern the beginnings of a distinction between these two elements, if we consider the matter further. As we have already observed (see pp. 92–3) the expected is, apart from other factors, pleasant in mental life, and the occurrence of the unexpected gives a certain shock, which tends to be slightly unpleasant. But as Groos has pointed out, there are occasions on which the shock of surprise appears as something attractive and is enjoyed accordingly.[1] The attraction found by the small child in the game of " Peep-Bo ", when an elder conceals himself behind something and suddenly reappears, must be in part due to the exciting character of this sort of shock. The attraction of a game such as dice, to take another example given by Groos,

[1] Groos, *Spiele des Menschen*, 204–5.

lies not only in the excitement of winning and losing,
but also in that of the alternation between expectation
and surprise at the decision of the throw. The surprise
must not be too violent. The sudden shock of a loud
noise, which is totally unexpected and wrenches the
attention away from its previous direction, causes acute
unpleasure, and this will prevent the rise of any other
feeling. Surprise is enjoyed when we are keyed up to
expect something interesting, but do not know the form
which it will take. It is in something of this frame of
mind that a child (or indeed an adult) goes to see fireworks,
with which it has little or no previous acquaintance. The
satisfaction that comes is in large measure due to the
exciting shock of the burst of light or flame and the
accompanying bang. We can distinguish this from the
sensory pleasure of the bright colours and lights. There is
in fact a distinction between pleasure and an excitement
of the self in which the conscious level appears as raised,
though the two may, as in this instance, occur together.

We have maintained that with the normal process of
life, including as it does a certain due alternation between
need or craving and its fulfilment, there goes a slight
constant feeling of pleasure, the stage of want and
striving being a necessary part of life. In normal health
and in normal conditions of life there is a feeling both of
pleasure as contrasted with unpleasure, and of the value
of a vividness and intensity of conscious life as contrasted
with apathy and dulness. The value of the sense of life
may be said to be due to both these factors. It can easily
be seen however that they do not always vary together.
It is possible owing to physical changes for the bodily
life to sink to a lower level of energy, to become apathetic
and dull. When a certain stage of self-consciousness
exists, the mind is able to struggle against this tendency
to depression, to the lower level of consciousness, regarding
it as something " bad " in comparison with the more vivid
life of alternation between desire and satisfaction. The
mere fact of apathy does not become unpleasant until there

is struggle against it. In the mere fact of resentment against monotony, a somewhat higher level is reached. But naturally this cannot be maintained without the material supplied by sensory stimulus. There may then be an intense wish for the stimulus of any sort of change. In a pathological case of apathy quoted by Sollier, we may quote a striking example. The patient, doubting of his own existence, spoke as follows : " I know well that these arms and legs must be mine, but I do not feel it." " He felt no pain and no pleasure," says Sollier, " and asked me to make him feel what they were, *especially pain*, in order to be able to feel that he lived."[1] What the man is longing for here is the vivid sense of life, and in the unpleasant experience of pain feels that there is a reaction in which this is attained more completely than in a pleasant experience. The state which we ordinarily know as boredom (*Langeweile, ennui*) shows much the same character. It arises when, owing to the absence of suitable objects and the fact that all essential needs are, somehow or other, easily supplied, the mind finds no ends to pursue. In such circumstances consciousness tends to sink to a lower level, to become apathetic and dull. Only when the self-consciousness is somewhat highly developed is there likely to be any struggle against this tendency. But when there is such an effort, we can see that it is directed, not so much towards obtaining pleasant experience, as towards obtaining experience which is vivid and exciting and may even include elements of unpleasure.

A distinction somewhat similar to the above meets us in the comparison between " play " and " earnest". In play, as we have already remarked, we feel ourselves free, and this gives it a certain value as compared with the more serious character of activity directed towards vital maintenance, in which there seems a certain measure of compulsion. Yet to give up one's life to nothing but play would in the general opinion be to sink to a lower level

---

[1] Sollier, *Le Mécanisme des Emotions*, 157. (Italics mine.)

of mental existence. To engage oneself in the serious business of maintenance of self and offspring, or to devote oneself whole-heartedly either to some ambition or to some altruistic end, is generally felt to mean a life of superior value to one devoted to play. The difference here perhaps is not so much in the acuteness of consciousness, as in the depth and energy with which the self is engaged where something of vital interest to itself is at stake. In this full and strenuous activity of the self we have a feeling of a value as compared with what appears as the superficiality and triviality of play, even though play may as a rule afford the additional interest of variety.

Perhaps the clearest form in which this same antithesis appears is in the experience of struggle and danger. In discussing the impulse to self-assertion we have already pointed out that in the experience of achieved mastery over external force there occurs a feeling of elation, which spreads its effects over the whole mental life. What we would here observe is that an element of heightened consciousness may also occur in the struggle itself, while it is still doubtful, and that in it there may be found an element of value not identical with the pleasure of success. In what is known as the spirit of adventure there are, I should judge, two factors : in the first place, the impulse towards novelty, away from the humdrum and expected, as that which tends to monotony ; in the second place, the desire to engage in a struggle which involves danger and so calls out the full energy of the self. In both ways there is sought an intensification of the conscious life, which appears as valuable, and especially in the fact of the dangerous struggle. In any more or less even contest the consciousness of self is heightened by the felt contrast of the force being exercised by the self with that being exercised by the opposition, and through awareness of the energy being exercised to meet the opposing force. And also, where there is danger and the intellect is sufficiently advanced to be able to realize the death or damage that is risked, the consciousness of life appears as height-

ened by the felt contrast of the sense of life with the
possible destruction or damage. There must indeed
be a certain degree of the emotion of fear. But fear if
at all strong will carry with it a sense of impotence and
a wish to escape from the danger, which would mean the
predominance of unpleasant feeling. The fear must
exist, but be transcended. Browning puts the following
words into Guido's mouth, expressing a certain exaltation
as he faces execution :

> You never know what life means till you die ;
> Even throughout life, 'tis death that makes life live,
> Gives it whatever the significance.
> For see on your own ground and argument,
> Suppose life had no death to fear, how find
> A possibility of nobleness
> In man prevented daring any more ?[1]

Schiller concludes thus his soldiers' song which praises
the fighting life :

> Und setzet Ihr nicht das Leben ein
> Nie wird Euch das Leben gewonnen sein.[2]

If you do not put your life to the hazard, you will never
win the full sense of life. Here is Martin Conway's
description of his first mountaineering danger, in which
we see how fear is present, even in the enhancement of
consciousness : " A strange agitation invaded all my
being. I was no doubt frightened and knew it, and
determined that no one else should know ; but there
was much more than terror, there was an extraordinary
exaltation such as Ulysses may have felt when he heard
the Sirens sing."[3]

We can see again how a certain division of mind exists
even in the remarkable description which the Russian
General Skobeleff gives of himself. " I believe that my
bravery is simply the passion and at the same time the

---

[1] *The Ring and the Book*, Guido's Second Speech, ll. 2375, etc.
[2] Schiller, " Wallenstein's Lager " (concluding lines).
[3] Martin Conway, *Mountain Memories*, 45.

contempt of danger. The risk of life fills me with an
exaggerated rapture. . . . A meeting of man to man, a
duel, a danger into which I can throw myself head foremost attracts me, moves me, intoxicates me. I am
crazy for it, I love it, I adore it. . . . When I throw
myself into an adventure in which I hope to find it, my
heart palpitates with the uncertainty ; I could wish at
once to have it appear and yet to delay. A sort of painful
and delicious shiver shakes me ; my entire nature runs to
meet the peril with an impetus which my will would in
vain try to resist."[1] In a lower form we can see the same
sort of attitude in the fascination with which the crowd
often watches dangerous performances such as tight-rope
walking, parachute descents, flying stunts. The onlookers
in some degree enter sympathetically into the experience
of the performer. Ordinary language recognizes here the
difference from the feelings of pleasure by its use rather
of such words as " thrill " or " excitement ". It is often
said that gambling is what for many ordinary persons in
our civilization gives an outlet for this spirit of adventure.
This is no doubt true, when anything is risked by the
gamble. But at the same time the sweepstake, in which
little is risked, is probably more popular even than
betting. The fascination of any sort of gambling perhaps
lies mainly in the opportunity it offers for hope, in the
varied possibilities which are opened up by the prospect
of winning, and the relief from the monotony of life
afforded thereby ; and the fact of the risks run is often
ignored. This is perhaps the case with the majority,
though others may enjoy the fact of the risks. By contrast with the life of danger and struggle there is often
ascribed to pleasure, as that which accompanies the
smoother and less impeded unfolding of capacities and
working out of conative trains, a certain inertness.
Dryden, writing at the end of the most disturbed period of
England's internal history, gives us some vigorous lines

---

[1] Quoted by James (*Varieties of Religious Experience*, 265) from an
article by Juliette Adam.

in which he expresses this semi-contempt for less strenuous times :

> Some lazy ages, lost in sleep and ease,
> No actions leave to busy chronicles ;
> Such whose supine felicity but makes
> In story chasms, in epochas mistakes,
> O'er whom Time gently shakes his wings of down,
> Till with his silent sickle they are mown.[1]

Probably many of the generation which went through the Great War have been inclined to take a certain pride in their experiences, and to ascribe a " supine felicity " to the preceding Victorian age. The value found in all such cases is not of course in the additional intensity of the pleasure *after* difficulties have been overcome, nor in the consciousness of a gradual and progressive attainment. It is found rather in the experience of the struggle itself, while it is still doubtful, and while the full energy of the self is called out in it. It will not be found if success is too easy, and it may exist even in the heroic losing struggle against odds. Doubtless characters vary and all cannot enter into this form of value. It is also probably the case that, even of those who can, it is only few who, like Skobeleff, are so attracted by the extremer forms of danger as to incur them voluntarily for their own sake. Most men do not incur serious danger for its own sake, but only incidentally to the pursuit of some other end conceived as of value, e.g. the satisfaction of the hunting impulse, the attainment of fame or power, or as a consequence of patriotic sentiment. Nevertheless we see that in pursuit of these ends another value may be incidentally obtained, and that probably, as in the case of pleasure, it may be all the more likely to be obtained, if not made directly the object of pursuit. This value, as the quotations given above should surely show, is to be defined as differing from pleasure. For the contrasting state is not so much unpleasure, as one of a lesser intensity and vividness of consciousness, which is felt to be lower in the scale of value.

[1] Dryden, " Astræa Redux."

As a result of the intensity of the conscious life, experienced especially in danger and perhaps in other exciting situations, there often seems to occur as a subsidiary effect an increase in the vividness of the ordinary accompanying sensations.   Martin Conway may be quoted again : " What would a man know about mountains who knew them only in days of cloudless peace ?   He that would enter into the treasures of the snows must wander in high places in Nature's many moods.   When the lightning is mated with the clouds, he must be a joyful onlooker and participant in the drama, even if he rejoice with trembling.   To climb along a narrow beclouded ridge when the gale sweeps across it and grasps at its crest, is a far more thrilling experience than to tread the slenderest arête in still air and clear sunshine.   A tower of ice whencesoever beheld will be a brilliant thing ; but the traveller who passes beneath one tottering to its fall will carry away a more vivid remembrance of its grandeur."[1] The following is recorded by Dr. R. W. McKenna in his book *The Adventure of Death* : " One soldier, a darkhaired Celt, had a very lively recollection of all the events which immediately preceded his first entry into the firetrench.   The prospect of facing danger had the effect of quickening all his faculties of perception, and he told me that, as he marched to the trenches, every blade of grass seemed to have become a more vivid green ; every wayside flower was clothed with a fresh beauty ; the warbling of the birds was sweeter than he had ever heard it before, and the little fleecy clouds in the sky were as white as driven snow."[2] No doubt an explanation of these facts on physiological lines may be brought forward. " That at times when strong emotion has excited the circulation to an exceptional degree, the clustered sensations yielded by surrounding objects are revivable with great clearness, often throughout life, is a fact noticed by

---

[1] Martin Conway, *Mountain Memories*, 58.
[2] McKenna, *The Adventure of Death*, 33.

writers of fiction as a trait of human nature."[1] We can
agree that there is truth in this, i.e. that a central excitation may exercise a diffused effect over the organism,
raising to a higher level many of the neural activities
occurring at the same time. But this of course does not
mean that a physiological explanation of the whole
phenomenon, which we have been describing, could be
accepted. The nature of the central excitation, that
which brings about the diffused effects, is the important
matter here. It is hardly possible to give an account
of this without bringing in a conative element, namely
the self-preservative effort of the conscious organism
and its reaction against that which appears to threaten
its existence.

A value may sometimes be found not only in struggle
and danger, but also in defeat and in suffering for which
there is no remedy. Unpleasure is in its nature an intenser
form of experience than pleasure, calling out more completely the energy of the self. But usually whatever
positive value may exist in this is outweighed by the negative value of the unpleasure. We can however make certain distinctions in regard to this according to the nature
and the temporal course of the experience. Any experience of unpleasure includes a reaction or resistance as an
element. In the case of purely physical unpleasure there
is the automatic reaction by the nervous elements primarily concerned. When any instinctive tendency is
frustrated, there is a conflict due to the persisting effort
of the tendency to fulfil itself against the impediment.
There is thus in the initial phase of any unpleasant
experience a factor of vividness or intensity, which
pleasure ordinarily does not possess. It would be going
too far to say that any value is ordinarily found in this
factor, for it is outweighed by the negative value of the
unpleasure. Where value will be found is rather in the
further course of the experience ; and that only where

---

[1] H. Spencer, *Principles of Psychology*, I, 235.

the self is fully engaged, e.g. in case of some physical suffering which the mind is able to conceive as a threat to the existence of the conscious self, or the frustration of some instinct into which the self enters deeply, such as sexual love, or a whole-hearted ambition. It is possible that the further course of such an experience may occur in one of two forms. Either in the first place the self may give way under the blow ; it may meet its onset with only the reaction of fear, and the effort of avoidance or escape, subsequently relapsing into an apathetic condition in which the level of the mental life is permanently lowered. In mere fear there is, to speak properly, no vigorous reaction by the self. There is rather a feeling as though the mind were being carried away by a force which it cannot resist. In such a series unpleasure and negative value will predominate. But on the other hand it is possible that the mind may meet the blow with courage and resist the tendency towards a mere depression. Such an attitude will involve a depth and intensity of mental reaction in which a value may be found outweighing the negative value of the unpleasure. And it may have the still further result of permanently energizing the mental life afterwards and calling out its capacities to the full extent, a result which would never have been attained if all had been constant success. John Marston in a famous prologue wrote :

> If any spirit breathe within this round
> Uncapable of weighty passion,
> As from his birth being hugged in the arms
> And nuzzled 'twixt the breasts of happiness.[1]

We may quote this too from Nietzsche : " The tension of soul in misfortune which communicates to it its energy, its shuddering in view of rack and ruin, its inventiveness and bravery in undergoing, enduring, interpreting, and exploiting misfortune, and whatever depth, mystery, disguise, spirit, artifice, or greatness has been bestowed

---

[1] Marston, Prologue to " Antonio's Revenge ".

upon the soul, has it not been bestowed through suffering, through the discipline of great suffering ? "[1]

In suffering a man's full nature is often first revealed to himself. " Nul ne se connait tant qu'il n'a pas souffert ", wrote A. de Musset.[2] Other valuable results can be ascribed to suffering and disappointment ; for instance, that they may purge the selfishness out of a man and leave him more open to the altruistic impulses, as Shakespeare makes Edgar say :

> A most poor man, made tame to fortune's blows
> Who by the art of known and feeling sorrows,
> Am pregnant to good pity.[3]

But of such further effects we are hardly speaking at present, but rather of the deepening and energizing of the soul's life in the mere act of being able to endure suffering without being crushed by it.

In the above there is given in effect a statement of what is at least a part of the æsthetic value of tragedy. Tragedy endeavours to recreate that form of intensity of experience through suffering, which may in real life also be found valuable, so that the onlooker may be able sympathetically to share in it. John Marston, in the prologue quoted above, was, it would seem, expressing this by the statement that only those who had experienced suffering themselves could enter fully into the meaning of tragedy.

> But if a breast
> Nailed to the earth with grief, if any heart
> Pierced through with anguish pant within this ring,
> If there be any blood whose heat is choak'd,
> And stifled with true sense of misery,
> They arrive most welcome.

There can hardly perhaps be a more striking example of a tragic emotion than the despair that comes with the realization that human life has no purpose and no

---

[1] Nietzsche, *Beyond Good and Evil*, 170.
[2] A. de Musset, " Nuit d'Octobre ".
[3] *King Lear*, Act IV, sc. 6.

meaning, as it is expressed in the famous outburst of Macbeth :

> Out, out, brief candle !
> Life's but a walking shadow, a poor player
> That struts and frets his hour upon the stage,
> And then is heard no more.   It is a tale
> Told by an idiot, full of sound and fury,
> Signifying nothing.

That there is value in this expression would be universally admitted, though it might seem strange and self-contradictory at first that value should be found in the recognition of non-value.   If we ask in what more nearly this value consists, the answer in the first place will be that it lies in the very depth and intensity of the despair. It is not merely an expression of the emptiness and purposelessness of life.   It is the expression of a mind which rebels with a supreme energy against that emptiness and against the lower level of effort and consciousness which might follow from its realization.   We see the reaction of a mind, which has hoped and willed intensely, to the realization that there is no value in life, while in this reaction it has in fact experienced the full power and energy of life.   At the same time, by the vividness of the expression of its feeling in metaphor or simile, it communicates its experience in a whole and complete character to others.

But with the foregoing we have hardly been adequate to the whole value in tragedy.   There seems to be a tragic value even when, so far as the characters depicted themselves are concerned, it is not possible to find any element of compensation for the suffering, when there is no point of their experience into which we wish to enter sympathetically.   For instance, we do not share sympathetically in the experiences of Ivan Karamazov, when Dostoievsky depicts him as losing his reason.   In so far as we were led to do so we could feel nothing but repulsion. In such cases value is found, I think, in so far as the writer is able to suggest to us some attitude in which we can contemplate the experience with a feeling which itself has value. If he can suggest to us some attitude of feeling which a universal mind, contemplating the facts, might be supposed to take, then in so doing we may be able in a sense to rise beyond the elements of non-value in the situation depicted. This is to " take upon us the mystery of things, As if we were God's spies " (as the famous speech in *King Lear* has it). There seem to me to be two elements of feeling in such an attitude, which may possess value. In the first place there may be pity felt for the victims of fate or disaster, into which there enters a colouring of tender emotion. The natural expression of this emotion is a tendency towards tears. The pity of course occurs in a " truncated " form ; i.e. there is no actual impulse to help or relieve, inasmuch as we have from the first taken a " make-believe " attitude, which affects all subsequent mental operations. With the emotions of pity and tenderness there is something of the value which is found in the exercise of these tendencies in real life. It is in this sort of feeling that we have that which is usually termed " pathos ". In the second place there may be an experience similar to that of the sublime. At first, in face of a world moved apparently by a power which is inscrutable to human judgments and does not conform to human standards, there is a tendency to abasement with fear. But then there may be something in the very mysteriousness of the power which attracts us. Being unknown it gives scope for wonder and speculation. We feel that it may be greater and juster than we see and it is not for us to judge it. " Shall mortal man be more just than God, shall a man be more pure than his maker ? "[1] So we feel we can in some degree give ourselves to that power or identify ourselves with it, thus rising beyond the initial abasement and fear. If there is to be any actual value of this character in a tragedy, it must contain, if no other element of redemp-

[1] Job iv. 17.

tion, at least some suggestion that the disaster or suffering is a result of laws which have some universal currency, even though we cannot altogether from our point of view see their justification. To recur, for instance, to the case of Ivan Karamazov, his madness may appear to us as the inexorable result of his intellectual detachment from reality, of his sceptical playing with the facts of life.

A value not unlike that described above is that which we often find in a " romantic " melancholy ; for example as we find it expressed in many Scottish and Irish folk songs with their tunes ; (the lilting chants of the Hebrides are a good example). We like these songs chiefly, as I think, because they express an emotion which by its depth and seriousness contrasts with the lighter and more trivial emotions of ordinary life ; they take us out of the commonplace. Especially do they express, together with grief, tender emotion in a profound and moving form.

In the foregoing we have been discussing differences in the form of experience, which can occur within a single mind. There are also differences between minds in the capacity for affective and emotional depth. We believe that in this respect human minds are capable of experiencing a value which animal minds are not capable of. A somewhat similar distinction can, I think, be drawn between the feelings of youth and of mature age. The difference arises as the result of intellectual factors in the following manner. With the growth of a store of memories the facts which we meet acquire an enlarged significance. Any experience which we come across, whether in real life or art, is capable of calling up memories of previous experiences and comparison with them. We thus can understand and enter into things more fully. The whole life becomes more fully charged with meanings.

> Every day my sense of joy
> Grows more acute, my soul, intensified
> By power and insight, more enlarged, more keen.

Browning puts these words into the mouth of his imaginary

Cleon, though he looks forward to the tragic fact that simultaneously there may be a beginning of the decay of the physical powers. There is moreover another factor. While the undeveloped mind no doubt feels intensely, its experiences are all much on the same level; for it has no sure standard of comparison. It tends to react with equal vehemence at all times. Mature age, realizing more clearly what is trivial and what is important, should be capable of treating the trivial as such and of feeling more intensely by comparison the full depth of that which is essential. It seems clearly right to say that in these ways experience gains in depth with age, and that so too there is a gain in felt value. A difference of the same sort, though much greater, exists, as we believe, between animal and human minds.

There are, I would suggest, two other dimensions, within which the functional side of mental life moves, in addition to those described above. But with neither of them does there appear to be feeling necessarily bound up, feeling, that is to say, in the sense of felt value. There is in the first place that form in which all conations occur, and which moves between degrees of tension and relaxation.[1] These terms are those which describe the varying form of the mental life during the temporal progress of a conation, i.e. its variation from energy and effort of pursuit to the terminating state of quiescence and completed satisfaction. The normal variation during the progress of a conation is from tension to relaxation. It is the common form which every conative process, including that of attention, tends to take. In itself it does not appear to carry with it any feeling in the form of value. We have pointed out already that the state of tension is not in itself unpleasant, nor does the state of relaxation, the final phase of a conative process, necessarily carry with it a

---

[1] In this I am to some extent following the views of Wundt, *Physiologische Psychologie*, II, 296–7 and 343–4, and those of Royce, *Outlines of Psychology*, 180.

feeling of value. Doubtless both tension and unpleasure
are at a high level when progress towards an end is held
up. But tension is also at a high level during the early
stages of any exercise for which there has been a craving,
and while the powers of the sense organs or the body
generally are still fresh and unexhausted. It changes
to a lower level as the impulse to exercise is worked out.
With this lower level of tension and activity we often
feel there is a lesser value. When relaxation is pleasant,
it is because fatigue has set in, and the activity, being
impeded by the fatigue conditions, has become unpleasant.
We have tried to set forth the reasons for this above.
They do not appear to lie in the tension-relaxation
series itself.

The second dimension to which we refer is that which
involves degrees of unity in the conative side of mental
life. There are states in which attention is divided and
distracted, and no concentration on one end takes place.
It is possible to perform two tasks at once, but this always
means some tendency to automatism in one of the performances and often in both. As we have already
observed, the periods of distraction or dissipation of
attention are also those of a lowered intensity of consciousness.[1] Consciousness reaches a higher level when there is
concentration, with all the mental powers, on the pursuit
of a single end. It would seem also that there cannot be
the consciousness of agency or self-direction, for example
in the control of sensory impulses by fixed principles or
rules, unless there is a high degree of unity in the mental
life. Thus unity of mental direction seems to be a condition of both the classes of value previously mentioned.
Nevertheless it is difficult to see how there can be a feeling
of value bound up directly with such a sense of mental
unity. The value would seem to reside in the further
effects which may follow in a highly developed mind as
the result of unity, and not in the unity or harmony

[1] See p. 58.

itself. Unity or harmony in itself can hardly be represented as a valuable end. It can be attained by exclusion as well as by inclusion. A completely harmonious and self-consistent mind might also be one very poor in content and very poor in energy, and as the general opinion would be, lacking in any true worth.

We conclude that there exist these two felt values arising from the degrees, firstly of self-direction, secondly of the energy and depth of the reaction by the self; and that, as feelings arising directly from the form of the mental life, they may be regarded as parallel to the feelings of pleasure and unpleasure. The forms of the conative life which we have mentioned must always be present, to a greater or less extent, in every mental state. The conative life is always proceeding more or less successfully, with more or less freedom from outside compulsion, with more or less depth and intensity. At all times therefore there is a certain blending of these forms, and it becomes natural to ask now in what way this blending takes place, and how it affects the felt value in the experience. This question has already been touched on, but not fully discussed.[1]

Many writers have considered that in some of the cases mentioned by us above we have examples of " mixed " feelings, i.e. mixtures or blendings of pleasure and unpleasure. Lehmann, who, with many other writers, holds that there are no feelings except pleasure and unpleasure, is of opinion that in such cases as the feeling of sublimity, the enjoyment of melancholy or the attraction felt in dangerous sports and adventures, there is a blending of pleasure and unpleasure. To take the last-mentioned example, he states that in these cases the danger, which in itself has an unpleasant feeling tone, is yet present throughout the experience as the constant condition that the satisfaction of overcoming may arise. Being present as the constant condition, the unpleasure

[1] Pp. 258–9.

of the danger blends with the pleasure of overcoming, so that a mixed feeling of pleasure and unpleasure is formed, in which the one element or the other will predominate, in so far as the danger is or is not being successfully overcome. Similarly in the other cases mentioned the unpleasure is present as a constant condition in order that the pleasure of overcoming or transcending it may arise.[1] From the standpoint we have now reached I think it is possible to see that, in as far as there is any blending or mixture in these cases, it affects that which we have called the *Bewusstseinslage*, the form of the mental life, not the feelings regarded as having value. Take again the example of the enjoyment of danger. If we are striving for some object, and meet with some opposition in which bodily danger is involved, our conation is, for the time being at least, unsuccessful, and this in itself would carry with it a feeling of unpleasure, the threat of bodily harm bringing an additional element of unpleasure. At the same time however the opposition, together with the threat of bodily harm, may call out a very intense reaction, claiming the full power of the conscious self ; and with this form of the mental life there is felt a heightened consciousness which has a high positive value. We can therefore say that the mental reaction, the subjective or functional side of the mental life, exhibits two forms simultaneously. It is impeded, working against a difficulty, while at the same time it reaches a high level of activity and intensity. We may therefore be right to speak of the mental life as subject to a blending of these two forms. What does not seem possible is that the mental life should exhibit a mixture of two forms, in so far as they belong to the same dimension and are therefore opposed as contradictories. It is not possible at the same time and in the same respect for a conation to be both successful and unsuccessful. Nor does it seem possible that the feeling state which may result from an

---

[1] See Lehmann, *Die Hauptgesetze des menschlichen Gefühlslebens*, 273–7.

admixture of the forms belonging to different dimensions should be a blend of positive and negative value, of goodness and badness. These would also appear to be contradictories, and, if elements of both co-exist in one mental system, their relation should be rather that of *plus* and *minus*. As we saw previously, the experimental evidence put forward to show that pleasure and unpleasure can blend seems very doubtful.[1] On *a priori* grounds we should be inclined to judge it impossible. And in looking at the class of facts now under discussion surely we find this confirmed. At any one moment either the negative value, i.e. unpleasure, involved in the situation of struggle and danger may predominate, or else, as in the quotations we have given above, the positive value of the exaltation of consciousness in adventure. It will follow that at any one moment the mind is likely either to accept or to reject the total situation. We shall conclude then that, while the attitude or form of the mental life, the *Bewusstseinslage*, may exhibit a blend, yet, in respect of feeling regarded as value, there can be no blending of what are in effect contradictories.

In this however we must guard ourselves against implying that there can be anything of the nature of a mathematical subtraction of values. The feeling, being a state of the self, appertains to the mental life taken in its wholeness. One unpleasant factor amidst a large number of otherwise pleasant ones may so infect the whole that the experience may lose its value. A single buzzing fly may ruin the enjoyment of a lazy afternoon in the garden with its many possible sources of pleasure. A single unpleasing element in a work of art is capable of spoiling the effect of the whole. On the other hand we must also refuse to admit that in the mere fact of the summation and concurrence of values a further value can emerge of any " higher " order than those of the separate value-moments. That this is the way in which there may arise value of

[1] See p. 258.

a different order than that involved in the satisfaction
of single impulses has been maintained by several writers,
e.g. by I. A. Richards.[1] According to this view value
arises from the satisfaction of any impulse or appetency,
and that is more valuable which satisfies more impulses
and involves the frustration of the lesser number of other
impulses. Impulses forward or interfere with each other
owing to our inborn constitution in numerous ways, of
the details of which we are largely ignorant.[2] A true
value (or the highest value) does not consist in the intensity of a momentary thrill of pleasure, but in the organization of the impulses belonging to a conscious experience
for " freedom and fulness of life ".[3] The poet is capable
of more valuable experience than other men because of
his superior power of ordering experience ; " impulses
which commonly interfere with one another and are
conflicting, independent, and mutually distractive, in
him combine into a stable poise."[4] In relation to this
view we take the position that neither the summation of
separate value-moments nor their organization can in
themselves create a new element of value of any higher
or different order. In the experience, for example, of a
luxuriously warm bath several different elements of
pleasure may co-exist, yet the whole experience remains
on the sensory level ; and so far as we can tell, the
different pleasures sum themselves, even if we cannot
calculate the result with any pretence to accuracy. We
have endeavoured to explain in our previous discussions
how elements of value other than pleasure can have arisen.
The possibility of a self-conscious personality in man
arose through the growth of intellectual power and foresight, giving an advantage in the struggle for existence,
and the possibilities inherent herein were developed
through relations to others both of combat and of co-
operation in society. It is obvious that the values going
with self-direction and with intensity of reaction are only

[1] See his work, *The Principles of Literary Criticism.*
[2] Op. cit., 47–51.   [3] Ibid., 132.   [4] Ibid., 243.

possible in as far as self-consciousness exists. It is only man who is capable of appreciating adequately the difference between self-originated action and that which is automatic and unpurposed, between a full activity of the self and that which is slight or trivial. The awareness of these differences can only be present even to the higher animals in a very rudimentary form. Man must believe that in these respects there are sources of value open to him which are not open to less-developed minds. These values may be felt as existing either in moments of specially intense consciousness or as a permanent and durable background to the mental life. The element of temporal duration has of course its importance. Other things being equal, a condition is more valuable in proportion as it endures more stably. We have no means of measuring the relative importance of duration and intensity, but both must count. In our lives stability is best secured by the organization of the mental life under some one master-sentiment. But in any case value can only exist for us in so far as it is actually felt ; otherwise it is non-existent. These values exist for us in so far as there is some actual feeling of the self as being raised to a higher power, when selfhood or personality is experienced as fuller and more intense.

There are no doubt occasions when a lower degree of consciousness appears to man as good, but this is because the higher degrees of mental activity have become fatiguing ; that is to say they are being impeded by the fatigue conditions and have therefore become unpleasant. The element of negative value may, and often does, at this stage outweigh the values going with a high level of consciousness. But this does not prove that the higher level of consciousness does not always carry with it elements of positive value.

It must be admitted that in all this we are dealing with a class of facts in which exact definitions are difficult, and in which there is room for much difference of individual opinion. The scheme given above must be regarded as somewhat tentative. What we often find is an unwilling-ness on the part of theorists to admit that the values actually recognized by men are exhaustively described in the terms pleasure and unpleasure. But at the same time difficulties are found in determining what the other values are. An attempt in this direction has been made in the foregoing. The chief point lacking in this is perhaps this, that it has given no adequate account of the peculiar value which is almost invariably ascribed to the altruistic impulse, to the experience of self-giving, as we have termed it. The value appears to be found in the mere impulse to self-giving itself, in the attitude in which the good of others is willed with the emotions of pity, tender-ness, etc., and not to be dependent on the actual success of the efforts made to help others.[1] A ground may be found for this value in a certain widening and enriching of the mental life. James has quoted some good remarks from Horwicz on the nature of self-love. " We may with confidence affirm that our own possessions in most cases please us better not because they are ours, but simply because we know them better, realize them more intimately, feel them more deeply. We learn to appreciate what is ours in all its details and shadings, while the goods of others appear to us in coarse outlines and rude averages. . . . On close examination we shall almost always find that a great part of our feeling about what is ours is due to the fact that we *live closer* to our own things and so feel them more thoroughly and deeply."[2] It is not so much that we judge our own performances or possessions superior to those of others. A good many people are biassed in the other direction. It is rather the case that our own things are known to us in a full and intimate way, and are more vivid to us than those of others, of which we have knowledge rather from outside ; and this applies to all our experiences, the whole of that inner life which it is impossible to share with others. There is no doubt that

[1] See p. 215.
[2] James, *Principles of Psychology*, I, 326–7.

in altruistic love there is some tendency towards over-passing this distinction. In love we are impelled towards a completer sympathy with others. If there is sympathy without love, we are content to realize their experiences from outside ; and while we enter into them by a sympathetic echo, there is still present the awareness that, as the experiences of others, they are not our immediate concern. In the altruistic impulse man is impelled, when there is in him a sympathetic echo of the feelings of others, to enter into them with something of the same intimacy, fulness, and closeness which pertain to his own immediate experiences. The same intimacy and fulness of knowledge can of course never be attained, but there is at least a striving towards it. In so far as this is possible, we see how it is that the unselfish person, taking a close and vivid interest in a greater number of experiences, seems to lead a fuller life than one who takes an interest in others purely from the outside, and whose life is by contrast poor and lacking in content. But though this is true, it is hardly sufficient to account for the special character of the feeling in altruistic love, for there appears to be a peculiar value felt in the mere act of self-giving, apart from the width and variety of the experiences involved. It is true also, as we have pointed out[1] already, that the full value of self-giving in love is only possible where there is a developed self-consciousness, and that it involves not a loss, but rather a deepening of the self-consciousness. But this of course does not constitute the essential value of the self-giving itself. All we can do is to repeat that it does not seem possible, within the limits of a psychology starting from the individual mind, to account for this felt value, nor for the special character of the negative value which may be felt, when there is consciousness of action in conflict with the altruistic impulse. Ethical theory in attempting to account for these facts would have to enter into considerations of a wider character, with which we cannot deal here.

[1] See pp. 196–8,

It now remains to ask what is the relation of the values now mentioned to action, whether it is the same in principle as that of pleasure and unpleasure. Pleasure and unpleasure, it is plain, can never constitute the sole motives to action. We can only attain the value of success by first having something else to aim at, though at a certain stage of intellectual development it is possible to guide and confirm our strivings by the idea of the value. Similarly, the feelings of self-direction and of the intensity of the conscious life only come to us in the first place when we are following what appear to be other ends, given by our innate constitution. But though this is the case at first, men can at a developed stage of intellect make these values themselves into ends. They can recognize the value of freedom and fulness of life and guide their actions accordingly. In certain cases at least it would seem that these values can be effective as the sole motives to action in a way which is not possible in the case of pleasure. Thus the motive for the control of the sensory desires of the body and the practice of asceticism has been for the most part the wish to maintain the consciousness of freedom and self-mastery.[1] This motive cannot exist of course unless the bodily desires are first in existence and have some urgency of appeal. But this does not mean that action cannot be motived solely by the idea of the value of self-control. Again a man may from discontent with the tameness of ordinary life seek the exciting thrill of danger. Here too the full force of the mental reaction cannot be experienced unless the threat of bodily harm, involved in the danger, appears as something to be avoided and combated, something from which there is an initial tendency to shrink with fear. The will would have no content in these cases without the existence of the unwilled and automatic bodily impulse towards self-preservation. At the same time the purpose in these cases is directed towards the achievement of a conscious

---

[1] Cf. the quotation from Iamblichus, given above, p. 67.

state conceived as valuable. There is however no new principle of action involved in this. We have shown, in dealing with the will to power,[1] how by insensible gradations there can emerge from the will to maintenance of conscious life a will to its intensification or improvement. In that case too the main end has become a valuable state of consciousness, sought because of its value, though of course it can only be attained through bringing about an objective situation, for example that which consists in dominance over external force. Again, if in monotonous circumstances a man seeks to avoid sinking to a lower conscious level through causing a change, no matter what, in his objective surroundings, he is directly seeking to attain a state of consciousness because more valuable than that which exists at present.

The essential form of all impulse to action is this : direction towards objective change, change of content, which will have for its result a subjective state possessing greater value than the present state. But there can be a difference in the relative prominence of these two factors, the subjective and the objective. In the primitive stages of mind the impulse is, for the agent, directed outwards, towards the objective change. It may be a sensory fact, which the agent strives to maintain or reject ; but this is in essence an object to a subject. As intellect develops with the power of abstraction and reflection, it becomes increasingly possible that the impulse should be directed towards the objective change as bringing about a more valuable conscious state of the acting subject. Take the case, so often discussed in this connection, of the desire for posthumous fame. It is quite possible for a man, in so far as he remains on an instinctive and unreflective level, to make posthumous fame, the admiration or respect of succeeding generations, his direct end, and to aim at bringing it about. He may think very little, if at all, of the satisfaction given by the assurance of later

[1] See pp. 120–3 and 218.

fame, which he himself will feel during his own life. But in so far as he reflects and thinks things out, he will necessarily see that that on which his impulse must terminate is the performance of certain work, the effectuation of certain objective change in his environment, which will yield him the present certainty that fame will come later. That is to say, his impulse will tend to terminate on the state of mind, valuable for himself, which he thus secures. It follows that in the more developed minds the impulse to action may take the form of a discontent with the present and the aim at a future state of the agent conceived as valuable. The dominant note of such a mind may thus tend to be one of discontent rather than of happiness, and it is possible that in this we have the explanation of pessimistic utterances, such as that of Goethe quoted above.[1] Here however a distinction must be made between altruistic and other actions. The form described above is that which action may tend to take, when it springs from an instinct directed towards the preservation or the good of the agent himself. Altruistic action, that which springs from an instinct directed towards the preservation or the good of others, must always remain in the main consciously directed outwards, having essentially objective reference. The end aimed at may be the valuable state of consciousness of another ; and at the more highly developed stage of mind there does seem to arise the tendency to a discontent with the present, and towards making the end of conduct consist in the attainment of some future ideal state for others; for one's society or for humanity. But these ends pursued for others are objective with regard to the agent himself. It is true that this devotion to ideals for others may bring about in fact a state of consciousness for the agent possessing high value. But if the main conscious end of such action were to become the valuable state of the agent's own consciousness, the state of mind attending the conduct would necessarily be self-contradictory.

[1] See p. 211.

It should hardly be necessary to add that in the fore-going there is no attempt to lay down what is "absolutely" valuable, nor indeed to discuss the question whether such a concept as " absolute value " is possible. All we have done is to attempt to describe what values are actu-ally recognized. Thus also we cannot by reference to any standard lay it down that one value is superior to another. We can only give the relative values as apparently recog-nized in practice by human minds. What we seem to find is that with the development of intellect additional sources of value arise, and it is therefore in respect of a greater sum of values that we can judge there to have been a possibility of progress for conscious life. At the same time too, it must be agreed, additional sources of negative value are created. For ideals can be formed, and the more distant and difficult of attainment the ideal, the less the likelihood of mental contentment.

INDEX